A NOTE TO ME

A 12-Week guide to being a better you.

Copyright © 2022 by Kruti St Helen

All rights reserved. No part of this book may be reproduced or used in any manner without written permission of the copyright owner except for the use of quotations in a book review. For more information, address: ksthelen@beucounsellingservice.com

FIRST EDITION

ISBN:

978-1-80227-442-4 (paperback)
978-1-80227-443-1 (eBook)

WWW.BEUCOUNSELLINGSERVICE.COM

DEDICATION

MY SON
For a moment I blinked
and you went from being a child
to a man.
You bought me so much joy.
You bought me so much tears,
but most of all you have given me
so many reasons
to be proud of you.
I love you now and forever more.

MY HUSBAND
To my best friend,
who keeps me sane
in my hour of need.
Who has wiped my tears.
Who has hugged me in my
darkest moments.
Who has seen me fail,
and kept me strong.
Who has loved me
in my despair.
To whom I am complete.
I love you more than you know.

ACKNOWLEDGEMENTS

I am grateful to each and every client who walks into my practice as I am aware of the resilience and determination that it takes to grow and develop. I salute your commitment to yourself.

I am grateful for the hard times that I have been through because without them I would not learnt, grown or developed my character and become the person I am today.

I am grateful to all the people who have supported and believed in me even when my self doubt got hold of me. Having good people around me has grounded me and lifted me when I needed the boost.

GRATITUDE

The word gratitude originates from the Latin word 'gratia' which means grace, graciousness, or gratefulness and in some shape or form gratitude encompasses all these meanings. Gratitude is about being thankful for what, we as individuals receive whether it is tangible or intangible. With gratitude, we are then able to acknowledge the goodness that we have in and around our lives.

By showing gratitude, we can affirm our beliefs that there are good things in the world that happen and that we are benefiting from them daily. This does not mean that our world is perfect, it is in fact acknowledging that our world is not perfect, but it encourages us to find precious gems within this imperfect world to be grateful for. So, in simple terms gratitude is taking the time to think about all the positive things in your life rather than ruminating on the negatives ones that surround you.

When a person has little, it can be somewhat easy to be grateful for things, however in the current world that we live in, where people in general have quite a lot, it can be harder to feel grateful. Therefore, if you want to feel gratitude, you must practice gratitude and must work at it on a daily basis. For example, remind yourself how luckily you are every day and be thankful for things that happen to you daily.

Being grateful and thankful on a regular basis has shown to reduce depression, lower blood pressure, increase energy levels and happiness and even prolong life. Showing gratitude increases the feel-good neuro-transmitters dopamine and serotonin and helps you to deflect the negative thoughts that you might be feeling.

There are many ways that you can practice gratitude and being thankful. You could do a vision board, which involves creating a visual mood board of everything you are grateful for and then placing this board somewhere in your home to remind yourself to be grateful every day. If this does not suit you, you could do a gratitude jar. This is where you write down on a piece of paper, whenever something good happens and put it in a jar. Then next time you are feeling down, give the jar a shake and pick out one slip of paper.

Whatever you decide to do why not celebrate your minor and major accomplishments and perform small acts of kindness and learn to appreciate the small things.

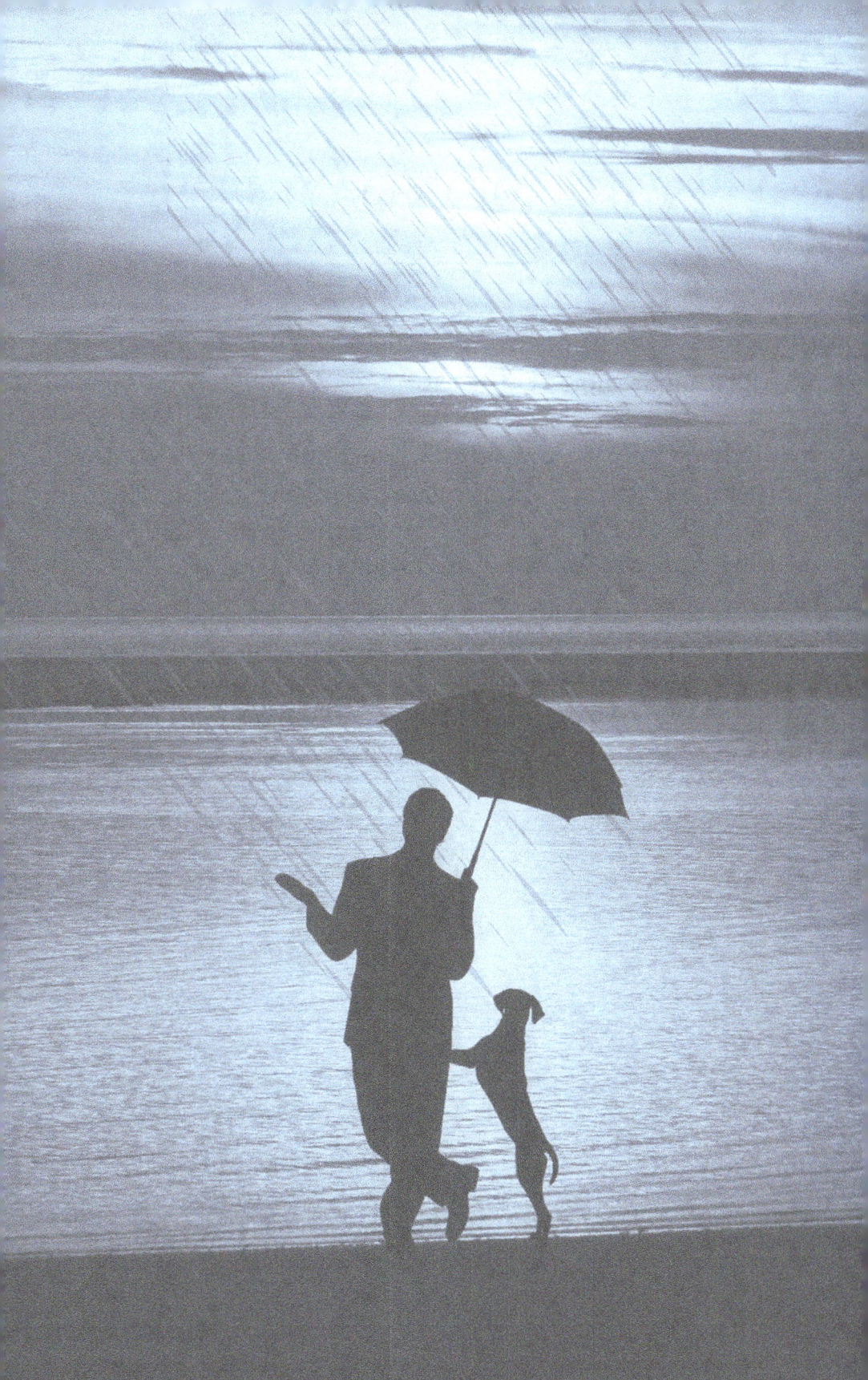

MONDAY

Morning Session

Find a quote, lyric, a picture, or something you have heard and stick it underneath. This is what you are going to start your day with! Make it funny or positive. Just as long as it makes you feel good. It is your dandelion in the concreate for the day!

Now write 5 goals that you want to achieve today. Remember you can make them small, medium or big, but make them achievable! Do not write things that you will not be able to achieve and whatever you cannot complete today does not roll over to tomorrow.

1. _____

   _____

2. _____

   _____

3. _____

   _____

4. _____

   _____

5. _____

   _____

Evening Session

Reflect on your day and now write 5 things or people that you are grateful for! Be Specific about your day. Remember you can be grateful for people, yourself or objects.

1. _____

   _____

2. _____

   _____

3. _____

   _____

4. _____

   _____

5. _____

   _____

Has it been a hard day? This is where you write 5 things or people you want to forgive. Again, do not forget to be specific about the day! And remember you can include yourself, people or objects.

1. _____

   _____

2. _____

   _____

3. _____

   _____

4. _____

   _____

5. _____

   _____

Reflection Space

This is your space! This is where you can make a few notes, you can do a spider diagram, you can doodle, or you can simply write down how you feel. If you are going to write down how you feel, remember to not rant and whine about your day, but to think of about, what you have learnt from the day and how you could improve for the next day. Ranting and moaning about the day will only create negative emotions and leave you feeling down. Keep it positive!

TUESDAY

Morning Session

Find a quote, lyric, a picture, or something you have heard and stick it underneath. This is what you are going to start your day with! Make it funny or positive. Just as long as it makes you feel good. It is your dandelion in the concrete for the day!

Now write 5 goals that you want to achieve today. Remember you can make them small, medium or big, but make them achievable! Do not write things that you will not be able to achieve and whatever you cannot complete today does not roll over to tomorrow.

1. _____

   _____

2. _____

   _____

3. _____

   _____

4. _____

   _____

5. _____

   _____

Evening Session

Reflect on your day and now write 5 things or people that you are grateful for! Be Specific about your day. Remember you can be grateful for people, yourself or objects.

1. _____

   _____

2. _____

   _____

3. _____

   _____

4. _____

   _____

5. _____

   _____

Has it been a hard day? This is where you write 5 things or people you want to forgive. Again, do not forget to be specific about the day! And remember you can include yourself, people or objects.

1. _____

   _____

2. _____

   _____

3. _____

   _____

4. _____

   _____

5. _____

   _____

Reflection Space

This is your space! This is where you can make a few notes, you can do a spider diagram, you can doodle, or you can simply write down how you feel. If you are going to write down how you feel, remember to not rant and whine about your day, but to think of about, what you have learnt from the day and how you could improve for the next day. Ranting and moaning about the day will only create negative emotions and leave you feeling down. Keep it positive!

WEDNESDAY

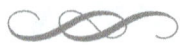

Morning Session

Find a quote, lyric, a picture, or something you have heard and stick it underneath. This is what you are going to start your day with! Make it funny or positive. Just as long as it makes you feel good. It is your dandelion in the concreate for the day!

Now write 5 goals that you want to achieve today. Remember you can make them small, medium or big, but make them achievable! Do not write things that you will not be able to achieve and whatever you cannot complete today does not roll over to tomorrow.

1. _____

   _____

2. _____

   _____

3. _____

   _____

4. _____

   _____

5. _____

   _____

Evening Session

Reflect on your day and now write 5 things or people that you are grateful for! Be Specific about your day. Remember you can be grateful for people, yourself or objects.

1. _____

   _____

2. _____

   _____

3. _____

   _____

4. _____

   _____

5. _____

   _____

   _____

Has it been a hard day? This is where you write 5 things or people you want to forgive. Again, do not forget to be specific about the day! And remember you can include yourself, people or objects.

1. _____

   _____

2. _____

   _____

3. _____

   _____

4. _____

   _____

5. _____

   _____

Reflection Space

This is your space! This is where you can make a few notes, you can do a spider diagram, you can doodle, or you can simply write down how you feel. If you are going to write down how you feel, remember to not rant and whine about your day, but to think of about, what you have learnt from the day and how you could improve for the next day. Ranting and moaning about the day will only create negative emotions and leave you feeling down. Keep it positive!

THURSDAY

Morning Session

Find a quote, lyric, a picture, or something you have heard and stick it underneath. This is what you are going to start your day with! Make it funny or positive. Just as long as it makes you feel good. It is your dandelion in the concrete for the day!

Now write 5 goals that you want to achieve today. Remember you can make them small, medium or big, but make them achievable! Do not write things that you will not be able to achieve and whatever you cannot complete today does not roll over to tomorrow.

1. _____

   _____

2. _____

   _____

3. _____

   _____

4. _____

   _____

5. _____

   _____

   _____

Evening Session

Reflect on your day and now write 5 things or people that you are grateful for! Be Specific about your day. Remember you can be grateful for people, yourself or objects.

1. _____

   _____

2. _____

   _____

3. _____

   _____

4. _____

   _____

5. _____

   _____

   _____

Has it been a hard day? This is where you write 5 things or people you want to forgive. Again, do not forget to be specific about the day! And remember you can include yourself, people or objects.

1. _____

_____

2. _____

_____

3. _____

_____

4. _____

_____

5. _____

_____

_____

Reflection Space

This is your space! This is where you can make a few notes, you can do a spider diagram, you can doodle, or you can simply write down how you feel. If you are going to write down how you feel, remember to not rant and whine about your day, but to think of about, what you have learnt from the day and how you could improve for the next day. Ranting and moaning about the day will only create negative emotions and leave you feeling down. Keep it positive!

FRIDAY

Morning Session

Find a quote, lyric, a picture, or something you have heard and stick it underneath. This is what you are going to start your day with! Make it funny or positive. Just as long as it makes you feel good. It is your dandelion in the concreate for the day!

Now write 5 goals that you want to achieve today. Remember you can make them small, medium or big, but make them achievable! Do not write things that you will not be able to achieve and whatever you cannot complete today does not roll over to tomorrow.

1. _____

   _____

2. _____

   _____

3. _____

   _____

4. _____

   _____

5. _____

   _____

   _____

Evening Session

Reflect on your day and now write 5 things or people that you are grateful for! Be Specific about your day. Remember you can be grateful for people, yourself or objects.

1. _____

_____

2. _____

_____

3. _____

_____

4. _____

_____

5. _____

_____

_____

Has it been a hard day? This is where you write 5 things or people you want to forgive. Again, do not forget to be specific about the day! And remember you can include yourself, people or objects.

1. _____

   _____

2. _____

   _____

3. _____

   _____

4. _____

   _____

5. _____

   _____

   _____

Reflection Space

This is your space! This is where you can make a few notes, you can do a spider diagram, you can doodle, or you can simply write down how you feel. If you are going to write down how you feel, remember to not rant and whine about your day, but to think of about, what you have learnt from the day and how you could improve for the next day. Ranting and moaning about the day will only create negative emotions and leave you feeling down. Keep it positive!

SATURDAY

Morning Session

Find a quote, lyric, a picture, or something you have heard and stick it underneath. This is what you are going to start your day with! Make it funny or positive. Just as long as it makes you feel good. It is your dandelion in the concreate for the day!

Now write 5 goals that you want to achieve today. Remember you can make them small, medium or big, but make them achievable! Do not write things that you will not be able to achieve and whatever you cannot complete today does not roll over to tomorrow.

1. _____

   _____

2. _____

   _____

3. _____

   _____

4. _____

   _____

5. _____

   _____

   _____

Evening Session

Reflect on your day and now write 5 things or people that you are grateful for! Be Specific about your day. Remember you can be grateful for people, yourself or objects.

1. _____

   _____

2. _____

   _____

3. _____

   _____

4. _____

   _____

5. _____

   _____

   _____

Has it been a hard day? This is where you write 5 things or people you want to forgive. Again, do not forget to be specific about the day! And remember you can include yourself, people or objects.

1. _____

   _____

2. _____

   _____

3. _____

   _____

4. _____

   _____

5. _____

   _____

Reflection Space

This is your space! This is where you can make a few notes, you can do a spider diagram, you can doodle, or you can simply write down how you feel. If you are going to write down how you feel, remember to not rant and whine about your day, but to think of about, what you have learnt from the day and how you could improve for the next day. Ranting and moaning about the day will only create negative emotions and leave you feeling down. Keep it positive!

SUNDAY

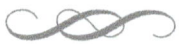

Morning Session

Find a quote, lyric, a picture, or something you have heard and stick it underneath. This is what you are going to start your day with! Make it funny or positive. Just as long as it makes you feel good. It is your dandelion in the concreate for the day!

Now write 5 goals that you want to achieve today. Remember you can make them small, medium or big, but make them achievable! Do not write things that you will not be able to achieve and whatever you cannot complete today does not roll over to tomorrow.

1. _____

   _____

2. _____

   _____

3. _____

   _____

4. _____

   _____

5. _____

   _____

   _____

Evening Session

Reflect on your day and now write 5 things or people that you are grateful for! Be Specific about your day. Remember you can be grateful for people, yourself or objects.

1. _____

_____

2. _____

_____

3. _____

_____

4. _____

_____

5. _____

_____

_____

Has it been a hard day? This is where you write 5 things or people you want to forgive. Again, do not forget to be specific about the day! And remember you can include yourself, people or objects.

1. _____

_____

2. _____

_____

3. _____

_____

4. _____

_____

5. _____

_____

Reflection Space

This is your space! This is where you can make a few notes, you can do a spider diagram, you can doodle, or you can simply write down how you feel. If you are going to write down how you feel, remember to not rant and whine about your day, but to think of about, what you have learnt from the day and how you could improve for the next day. Ranting and moaning about the day will only create negative emotions and leave you feeling down. Keep it positive!

POSITIVE THOUGHTS

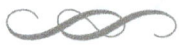

Each day is a new day and a new beginning to seize opportunities that may come our way. We can either be open to those opportunities or we can close ourselves to what could be!

To seize these opportunities, as little as they may be, we need to change our mind set. If we look at the world with a grim view, then all we will see is the darkness that stares back at us, but if we were to open our eyes and see the dandelions amongst the concrete then we might actually start to see that the world is not a bad place!

There are plenty of reasons why thinking positively can help you and although thinking positively will not solve your problems, it will make it managable.

Thinking positively can help you to push forward in your day and can help you to encourage overwhelming obstacles that you may have thought to be difficult and had to overcome. It can make you believe that you can get what you want, and it can motivate you into achieving things that you thought would not be possible.

Positive thinking can be done using various techniques that can be proved effective. Starting every morning with something positive that can be uplifting or encouraging can help you brighten your mood each day.

When learning to think positive, it is important to teach yourself to talk positively. This is about being kind to yourself and being patience with yourself. Research shows that just a small shift in how you talk to yourself can influence your ability to regulate your feelings, thoughts, and behaviours.

To create positive thoughts, it is important to surround yourself with positive people. Being around positive people can help improve your self-esteem and can increase your chances of reaching your goals.

It is important to remember that when you are practicing positivity that you give yourself time and be patience with yourself. You will not learn to become an optimist overnight, but eventually with practice, you will soon learn self-acceptance and will learn to be less critical.

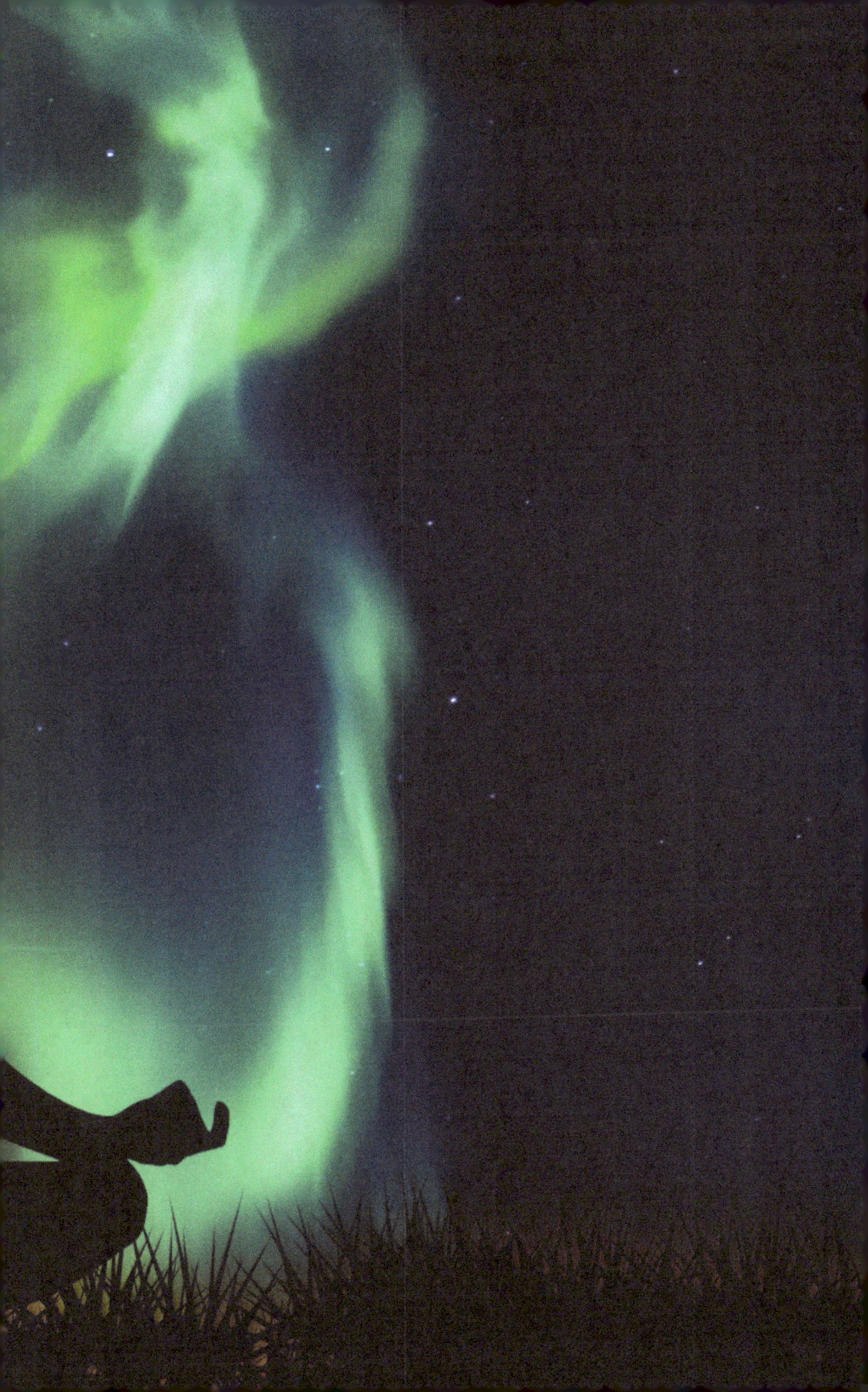

MONDAY

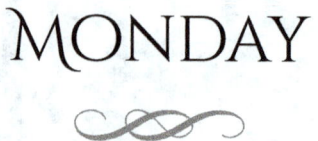

Morning Session

Find a quote, lyric, a picture, or something you have heard and stick it underneath. This is what you are going to start your day with! Make it funny or positive. Just as long as it makes you feel good. It is your dandelion in the concreate for the day!

Now write 5 goals that you want to achieve today. Remember you can make them small, medium or big, but make them achievable! Do not write things that you will not be able to achieve and whatever you cannot complete today does not roll over to tomorrow.

1. _____

   _____

2. _____

   _____

3. _____

   _____

4. _____

   _____

5. _____

   _____

Evening Session

Reflect on your day and now write 5 things or people that you are grateful for! Be Specific about your day. Remember you can be grateful for people, yourself or objects.

1. _____

   _____

2. _____

   _____

3. _____

   _____

4. _____

   _____

5. _____

   _____

Has it been a hard day? This is where you write 5 things or people you want to forgive. Again, do not forget to be specific about the day! And remember you can include yourself, people or objects.

1. _____

   _____

2. _____

   _____

3. _____

   _____

4. _____

   _____

5. _____

   _____

   _____

Reflection Space

This is your space! This is where you can make a few notes, you can do a spider diagram, you can doodle, or you can simply write down how you feel. If you are going to write down how you feel, remember to not rant and whine about your day, but to think of about, what you have learnt from the day and how you could improve for the next day. Ranting and moaning about the day will only create negative emotions and leave you feeling down. Keep it positive!

TUESDAY

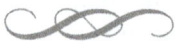

Morning Session

Find a quote, lyric, a picture, or something you have heard and stick it underneath. This is what you are going to start your day with! Make it funny or positive. Just as long as it makes you feel good. It is your dandelion in the concreate for the day!

Now write 5 goals that you want to achieve today. Remember you can make them small, medium or big, but make them achievable! Do not write things that you will not be able to achieve and whatever you cannot complete today does not roll over to tomorrow.

1. _____

   _____

2. _____

   _____

3. _____

   _____

4. _____

   _____

5. _____

   _____

   _____

Evening Session

Reflect on your day and now write 5 things or people that you are grateful for! Be Specific about your day. Remember you can be grateful for people, yourself or objects.

1. _____

_____

2. _____

_____

3. _____

_____

4. _____

_____

5. _____

_____

_____

Has it been a hard day? This is where you write 5 things or people you want to forgive. Again, do not forget to be specific about the day! And remember you can include yourself, people or objects.

1. _____
   _____

2. _____
   _____

3. _____
   _____

4. _____
   _____

5. _____
   _____

Reflection Space

This is your space! This is where you can make a few notes, you can do a spider diagram, you can doodle, or you can simply write down how you feel. If you are going to write down how you feel, remember to not rant and whine about your day, but to think of about, what you have learnt from the day and how you could improve for the next day. Ranting and moaning about the day will only create negative emotions and leave you feeling down. Keep it positive!

WEDNESDAY

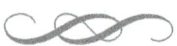

Morning Session

Find a quote, lyric, a picture, or something you have heard and stick it underneath. This is what you are going to start your day with! Make it funny or positive. Just as long as it makes you feel good. It is your dandelion in the concreate for the day!

Now write 5 goals that you want to achieve today. Remember you can make them small, medium or big, but make them achievable! Do not write things that you will not be able to achieve and whatever you cannot complete today does not roll over to tomorrow.

1. _____

   _____

2. _____

   _____

3. _____

   _____

4. _____

   _____

5. _____

   _____

Evening Session

Reflect on your day and now write 5 things or people that you are grateful for! Be Specific about your day. Remember you can be grateful for people, yourself or objects.

1. _____

_____

2. _____

_____

3. _____

_____

4. _____

_____

5. _____

_____

_____

Has it been a hard day? This is where you write 5 things or people you want to forgive. Again, do not forget to be specific about the day! And remember you can include yourself, people or objects.

1. _____
   _____

2. _____
   _____

3. _____
   _____

4. _____
   _____

5. _____
   _____

Reflection Space

This is your space! This is where you can make a few notes, you can do a spider diagram, you can doodle, or you can simply write down how you feel. If you are going to write down how you feel, remember to not rant and whine about your day, but to think of about, what you have learnt from the day and how you could improve for the next day. Ranting and moaning about the day will only create negative emotions and leave you feeling down. Keep it positive!

THURSDAY

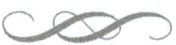

Morning Session

Find a quote, lyric, a picture, or something you have heard and stick it underneath. This is what you are going to start your day with! Make it funny or positive. Just as long as it makes you feel good. It is your dandelion in the concreate for the day!

Now write 5 goals that you want to achieve today. Remember you can make them small, medium or big, but make them achievable! Do not write things that you will not be able to achieve and whatever you cannot complete today does not roll over to tomorrow.

1. _____

   _____

2. _____

   _____

3. _____

   _____

4. _____

   _____

5. _____

   _____

   _____

Evening Session

Reflect on your day and now write 5 things or people that you are grateful for! Be Specific about your day. Remember you can be grateful for people, yourself or objects.

1. _____

_____

2. _____

_____

3. _____

_____

4. _____

_____

5. _____

_____

Has it been a hard day? This is where you write 5 things or people you want to forgive. Again, do not forget to be specific about the day! And remember you can include yourself, people or objects.

1. _____

   _____

2. _____

   _____

3. _____

   _____

4. _____

   _____

5. _____

   _____

   _____

Reflection Space

This is your space! This is where you can make a few notes, you can do a spider diagram, you can doodle, or you can simply write down how you feel. If you are going to write down how you feel, remember to not rant and whine about your day, but to think of about, what you have learnt from the day and how you could improve for the next day. Ranting and moaning about the day will only create negative emotions and leave you feeling down. Keep it positive!

FRIDAY

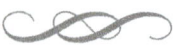

Morning Session

Find a quote, lyric, a picture, or something you have heard and stick it underneath. This is what you are going to start your day with! Make it funny or positive. Just as long as it makes you feel good. It is your dandelion in the concreate for the day!

Now write 5 goals that you want to achieve today. Remember you can make them small, medium or big, but make them achievable! Do not write things that you will not be able to achieve and whatever you cannot complete today does not roll over to tomorrow.

1. _____

_____

2. _____

_____

3. _____

_____

4. _____

_____

5. _____

_____

_____

Evening Session

Reflect on your day and now write 5 things or people that you are grateful for! Be Specific about your day. Remember you can be grateful for people, yourself or objects.

1. _____

_____

2. _____

_____

3. _____

_____

4. _____

_____

5. _____

_____

_____

Has it been a hard day? This is where you write 5 things or people you want to forgive. Again, do not forget to be specific about the day! And remember you can include yourself, people or objects.

1. _____
   _____

2. _____
   _____

3. _____
   _____

4. _____
   _____

5. _____
   _____
   _____

Reflection Space

This is your space! This is where you can make a few notes, you can do a spider diagram, you can doodle, or you can simply write down how you feel. If you are going to write down how you feel, remember to not rant and whine about your day, but to think of about, what you have learnt from the day and how you could improve for the next day. Ranting and moaning about the day will only create negative emotions and leave you feeling down. Keep it positive!

SATURDAY

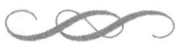

Morning Session

Find a quote, lyric, a picture, or something you have heard and stick it underneath. This is what you are going to start your day with! Make it funny or positive. Just as long as it makes you feel good. It is your dandelion in the concreate for the day!

Now write 5 goals that you want to achieve today. Remember you can make them small, medium or big, but make them achievable! Do not write things that you will not be able to achieve and whatever you cannot complete today does not roll over to tomorrow.

1. _____

   _____

2. _____

   _____

3. _____

   _____

4. _____

   _____

5. _____

   _____

   _____

Evening Session

Reflect on your day and now write 5 things or people that you are grateful for! Be Specific about your day. Remember you can be grateful for people, yourself or objects.

1. _____

_____

2. _____

_____

3. _____

_____

4. _____

_____

5. _____

_____

_____

Has it been a hard day? This is where you write 5 things or people you want to forgive. Again, do not forget to be specific about the day! And remember you can include yourself, people or objects.

1. _____

   _____

2. _____

   _____

3. _____

   _____

4. _____

   _____

5. _____

   _____

   _____

Reflection Space

This is your space! This is where you can make a few notes, you can do a spider diagram, you can doodle, or you can simply write down how you feel. If you are going to write down how you feel, remember to not rant and whine about your day, but to think of about, what you have learnt from the day and how you could improve for the next day. Ranting and moaning about the day will only create negative emotions and leave you feeling down. Keep it positive!

SUNDAY

Morning Session

Find a quote, lyric, a picture, or something you have heard and stick it underneath. This is what you are going to start your day with! Make it funny or positive. Just as long as it makes you feel good. It is your dandelion in the concreate for the day!

Now write 5 goals that you want to achieve today. Remember you can make them small, medium or big, but make them achievable! Do not write things that you will not be able to achieve and whatever you cannot complete today does not roll over to tomorrow.

1. _____

   _____

2. _____

   _____

3. _____

   _____

4. _____

   _____

5. _____

   _____

Evening Session

Reflect on your day and now write 5 things or people that you are grateful for! Be Specific about your day. Remember you can be grateful for people, yourself or objects.

1. _____

   _____

2. _____

   _____

3. _____

   _____

4. _____

   _____

5. _____

   _____

Has it been a hard day? This is where you write 5 things or people you want to forgive. Again, do not forget to be specific about the day! And remember you can include yourself, people or objects.

1. _____

   _____

2. _____

   _____

3. _____

   _____

4. _____

   _____

5. _____

   _____

   _____

Reflection Space

This is your space! This is where you can make a few notes, you can do a spider diagram, you can doodle, or you can simply write down how you feel. If you are going to write down how you feel, remember to not rant and whine about your day, but to think of about, what you have learnt from the day and how you could improve for the next day. Ranting and moaning about the day will only create negative emotions and leave you feeling down. Keep it positive!

PHYSICAL EXERCISE

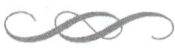

When thinking about physical exercise, we think about it in terms of getting fitter, leaner, and losing weight, however exercising can also be particularly good for your mental wellbeing. Regular exercise can have a huge positive impact on depression, anxiety, stress, and memory.

Various research has shown that participants felt more content, awake and calmer after being active compared to being inactive and found a greater improvement in their mood and in their sleep.

When we exercise, our brain releases endorphins. These are the neurotransmitters of the brain. The endorphins are produced to relieve stress and pain and can produce the same feeling of euphoria as the class of drugs, opioids. Not only does exercising produce endorphins, but physical exercise also produces dopamine, norepinephrine, and serotonin which all play an important part in regulating your mood.

The great thing about being active is that you do not have to do this, being stuck is a gym sweating away. There are so many ways that you can introduce physical activity into your life. At a considerably basic level, physical exercising means moving your body so going for a walk, a run, a swim, or even skipping with a rope would all include this.

However, in a busy life, it can be hard to find and maintain physical activity in your daily life, so why not try to incorporate it into your everyday life. Take the stairs instead of the lift or walk your kids to school instead of driving or join a sports team as this can be a fun and interactive way of exercising.

Whatever you do, make physical exercise a fun, daily and interactive part of your life. It is important to not allow it to become a chore and to include it in your everyday life. This way you are more likely to stick to it and reap the benefits from it rather than seeing it as another thing to do or complete in the day.

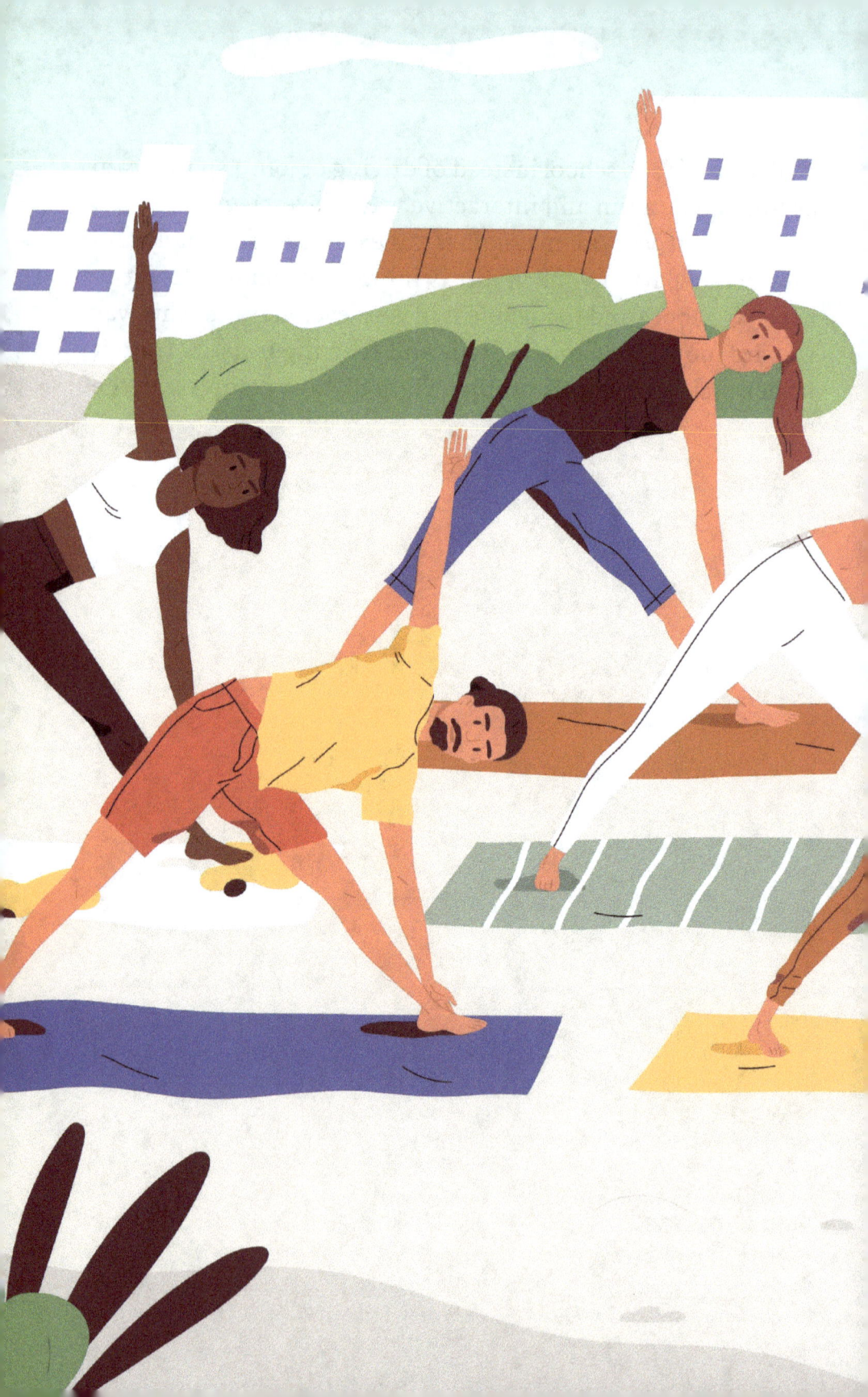

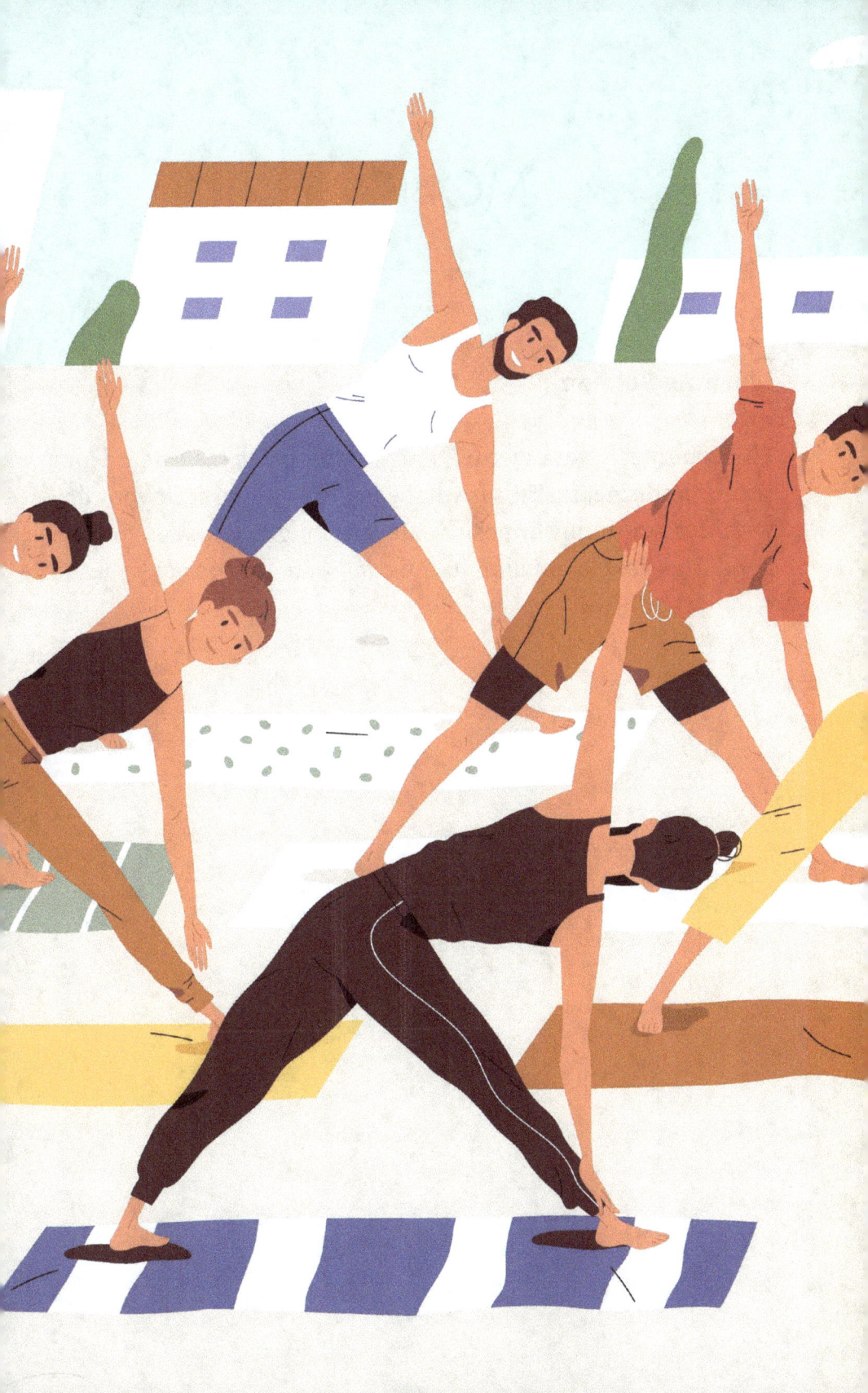

MONDAY

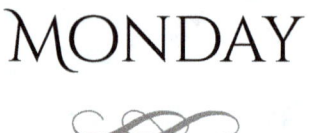

Morning Session

Find a quote, lyric, a picture, or something you have heard and stick it underneath. This is what you are going to start your day with! Make it funny or positive. Just as long as it makes you feel good. It is your dandelion in the concreate for the day!

Now write 5 goals that you want to achieve today. Remember you can make them small, medium or big, but make them achievable! Do not write things that you will not be able to achieve and whatever you cannot complete today does not roll over to tomorrow.

1. _____

   _____

2. _____

   _____

3. _____

   _____

4. _____

   _____

5. _____

   _____

Evening Session

Reflect on your day and now write 5 things or people that you are grateful for! Be Specific about your day. Remember you can be grateful for people, yourself or objects.

1. _____

_____

2. _____

_____

3. _____

_____

4. _____

_____

5. _____

_____

Has it been a hard day? This is where you write 5 things or people you want to forgive. Again, do not forget to be specific about the day! And remember you can include yourself, people or objects.

1. _____

   _____

2. _____

   _____

3. _____

   _____

4. _____

   _____

5. _____

   _____

   _____

Reflection Space

This is your space! This is where you can make a few notes, you can do a spider diagram, you can doodle, or you can simply write down how you feel. If you are going to write down how you feel, remember to not rant and whine about your day, but to think of about, what you have learnt from the day and how you could improve for the next day. Ranting and moaning about the day will only create negative emotions and leave you feeling down. Keep it positive!

TUESDAY

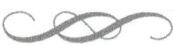

Morning Session

Find a quote, lyric, a picture, or something you have heard and stick it underneath. This is what you are going to start your day with! Make it funny or positive. Just as long as it makes you feel good. It is your dandelion in the concreate for the day!

Now write 5 goals that you want to achieve today. Remember you can make them small, medium or big, but make them achievable! Do not write things that you will not be able to achieve and whatever you cannot complete today does not roll over to tomorrow.

1. _____

   _____

2. _____

   _____

3. _____

   _____

4. _____

   _____

5. _____

   _____

Evening Session

Reflect on your day and now write 5 things or people that you are grateful for! Be Specific about your day. Remember you can be grateful for people, yourself or objects.

1. _____

   _____

2. _____

   _____

3. _____

   _____

4. _____

   _____

5. _____

   _____

Has it been a hard day? This is where you write 5 things or people you want to forgive. Again, do not forget to be specific about the day! And remember you can include yourself, people or objects.

1. _____

   _____

2. _____

   _____

3. _____

   _____

4. _____

   _____

5. _____

   _____

Reflection Space

This is your space! This is where you can make a few notes, you can do a spider diagram, you can doodle, or you can simply write down how you feel. If you are going to write down how you feel, remember to not rant and whine about your day, but to think of about, what you have learnt from the day and how you could improve for the next day. Ranting and moaning about the day will only create negative emotions and leave you feeling down. Keep it positive!

WEDNESDAY

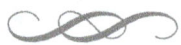

Morning Session

Find a quote, lyric, a picture, or something you have heard and stick it underneath. This is what you are going to start your day with! Make it funny or positive. Just as long as it makes you feel good. It is your dandelion in the concreate for the day!

Now write 5 goals that you want to achieve today. Remember you can make them small, medium or big, but make them achievable! Do not write things that you will not be able to achieve and whatever you cannot complete today does not roll over to tomorrow.

1. _____

   _____

2. _____

   _____

3. _____

   _____

4. _____

   _____

5. _____

   _____

Evening Session

Reflect on your day and now write 5 things or people that you are grateful for! Be Specific about your day. Remember you can be grateful for people, yourself or objects.

1. _____

   _____

2. _____

   _____

3. _____

   _____

4. _____

   _____

5. _____

   _____

Has it been a hard day? This is where you write 5 things or people you want to forgive. Again, do not forget to be specific about the day! And remember you can include yourself, people or objects.

1. _____

   _____

2. _____

   _____

3. _____

   _____

4. _____

   _____

5. _____

   _____

Reflection Space

This is your space! This is where you can make a few notes, you can do a spider diagram, you can doodle, or you can simply write down how you feel. If you are going to write down how you feel, remember to not rant and whine about your day, but to think of about, what you have learnt from the day and how you could improve for the next day. Ranting and moaning about the day will only create negative emotions and leave you feeling down. Keep it positive!

THURSDAY

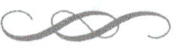

Morning Session

Find a quote, lyric, a picture, or something you have heard and stick it underneath. This is what you are going to start your day with! Make it funny or positive. Just as long as it makes you feel good. It is your dandelion in the concreate for the day!

Now write 5 goals that you want to achieve today. Remember you can make them small, medium or big, but make them achievable! Do not write things that you will not be able to achieve and whatever you cannot complete today does not roll over to tomorrow.

1. _____

   _____

2. _____

   _____

3. _____

   _____

4. _____

   _____

5. _____

   _____

Evening Session

Reflect on your day and now write 5 things or people that you are grateful for! Be Specific about your day. Remember you can be grateful for people, yourself or objects.

1. _____

   _____

2. _____

   _____

3. _____

   _____

4. _____

   _____

5. _____

   _____

Has it been a hard day? This is where you write 5 things or people you want to forgive. Again, do not forget to be specific about the day! And remember you can include yourself, people or objects.

1. _____

   _____

2. _____

   _____

3. _____

   _____

4. _____

   _____

5. _____

   _____

Reflection Space

This is your space! This is where you can make a few notes, you can do a spider diagram, you can doodle, or you can simply write down how you feel. If you are going to write down how you feel, remember to not rant and whine about your day, but to think of about, what you have learnt from the day and how you could improve for the next day. Ranting and moaning about the day will only create negative emotions and leave you feeling down. Keep it positive!

FRIDAY

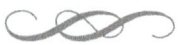

Morning Session

Find a quote, lyric, a picture, or something you have heard and stick it underneath. This is what you are going to start your day with! Make it funny or positive. Just as long as it makes you feel good. It is your dandelion in the concreate for the day!

Now write 5 goals that you want to achieve today. Remember you can make them small, medium or big, but make them achievable! Do not write things that you will not be able to achieve and whatever you cannot complete today does not roll over to tomorrow.

1. _____

   _____

2. _____

   _____

3. _____

   _____

4. _____

   _____

5. _____

   _____

Evening Session

Reflect on your day and now write 5 things or people that you are grateful for! Be Specific about your day. Remember you can be grateful for people, yourself or objects.

1. _____

_____

2. _____

_____

3. _____

_____

4. _____

_____

5. _____

_____

Has it been a hard day? This is where you write 5 things or people you want to forgive. Again, do not forget to be specific about the day! And remember you can include yourself, people or objects.

1. _____

   _____

2. _____

   _____

3. _____

   _____

4. _____

   _____

5. _____

   _____

Reflection Space

This is your space! This is where you can make a few notes, you can do a spider diagram, you can doodle, or you can simply write down how you feel. If you are going to write down how you feel, remember to not rant and whine about your day, but to think of about, what you have learnt from the day and how you could improve for the next day. Ranting and moaning about the day will only create negative emotions and leave you feeling down. Keep it positive!

SATURDAY

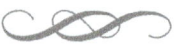

Morning Session

Find a quote, lyric, a picture, or something you have heard and stick it underneath. This is what you are going to start your day with! Make it funny or positive. Just as long as it makes you feel good. It is your dandelion in the concrete for the day!

Now write 5 goals that you want to achieve today. Remember you can make them small, medium or big, but make them achievable! Do not write things that you will not be able to achieve and whatever you cannot complete today does not roll over to tomorrow.

1. _____

   _____

2. _____

   _____

3. _____

   _____

4. _____

   _____

5. _____

   _____

Morning Session

Reflect on your day and now write 5 things or people that you are grateful for! Be Specific about your day. Remember you can be grateful for people, yourself or objects.

1. _____

   _____

2. _____

   _____

3. _____

   _____

4. _____

   _____

5. _____

   _____

Has it been a hard day? This is where you write 5 things or people you want to forgive. Again, do not forget to be specific about the day! And remember you can include yourself, people or objects.

1. _____

_____

2. _____

_____

3. _____

_____

4. _____

_____

5. _____

_____

Reflection Space

This is your space! This is where you can make a few notes, you can do a spider diagram, you can doodle, or you can simply write down how you feel. If you are going to write down how you feel, remember to not rant and whine about your day, but to think of about, what you have learnt from the day and how you could improve for the next day. Ranting and moaning about the day will only create negative emotions and leave you feeling down. Keep it positive!

SUNDAY

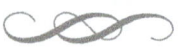

Morning Session

Find a quote, lyric, a picture, or something you have heard and stick it underneath. This is what you are going to start your day with! Make it funny or positive. Just as long as it makes you feel good. It is your dandelion in the concreate for the day!

Now write 5 goals that you want to achieve today. Remember you can make them small, medium or big, but make them achievable! Do not write things that you will not be able to achieve and whatever you cannot complete today does not roll over to tomorrow.

1. _____

   _____

2. _____

   _____

3. _____

   _____

4. _____

   _____

5. _____

   _____

Evening Session

Reflect on your day and now write 5 things or people that you are grateful for! Be Specific about your day. Remember you can be grateful for people, yourself or objects.

1. _____

_____

2. _____

_____

3. _____

_____

4. _____

_____

5. _____

_____

Has it been a hard day? This is where you write 5 things or people you want to forgive. Again, do not forget to be specific about the day! And remember you can include yourself, people or objects.

1. _____

   _____

2. _____

   _____

3. _____

   _____

4. _____

   _____

5. _____

   _____

Reflection Space

This is your space! This is where you can make a few notes, you can do a spider diagram, you can doodle, or you can simply write down how you feel. If you are going to write down how you feel, remember to not rant and whine about your day, but to think of about, what you have learnt from the day and how you could improve for the next day. Ranting and moaning about the day will only create negative emotions and leave you feeling down. Keep it positive!

MEDITATION

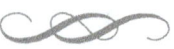

Meditation has been around for many years. Originally it was used to deepen ones understanding about life and to give great insight, however over the years the use of meditation has changed somewhat. Now a days we tend to use mediatation to relieve stress and anxiety in everyday life.

There have been various studies in recent years that have produced good evidence showing that meditation helps relieve participants of anxiety and depression, improves attention and concentration, and overall improves an individual's emotional wellbeing.

Living in a busy society can be very chaotic and can be non-stop and therefore it is easy to pick up bad habits by gathering up negative thoughts and feelings and hold on to them.

Spending just a few minutes of meditation every day can help restore your calm and inner peace and the beauty of meditation is that it is simple and inexpensive, and it does not require any equipment.

Meditation can encourage you to slow down and allow for a deeper self-reflection which can help you to discover positive attributes about yourself. It can also increase your self-awareness by allowing you to reflect on your thoughts and feelings without judging yourself, which in turn would improve your self-esteem.

With meditation you can practice it wherever you are, whether it is in short bursts or for a longer period. You can

practice it when you go out for a walk, eating, during a meeting and even while you are commuting.
Through meditation, we can train our minds to rewire our thoughts into more positive ones and eliminate the negative thoughts. Thus, causing mediation to have huge, long lasting benefits. I have included a short breathing exercising down below for you to try.

1. Relax your neck and shoulders. Close your eyes.
2. Keeping your mouth closed, take a deep breath through your nose. Notice how your chest inflates with air when you take the air in.
3. Breathe out slowly by blowing air through your mouth. Noticing your chest deflate from the air leaving.
4. Repeat this for 10 times and with each breath imagine your body sinking and relaxing.

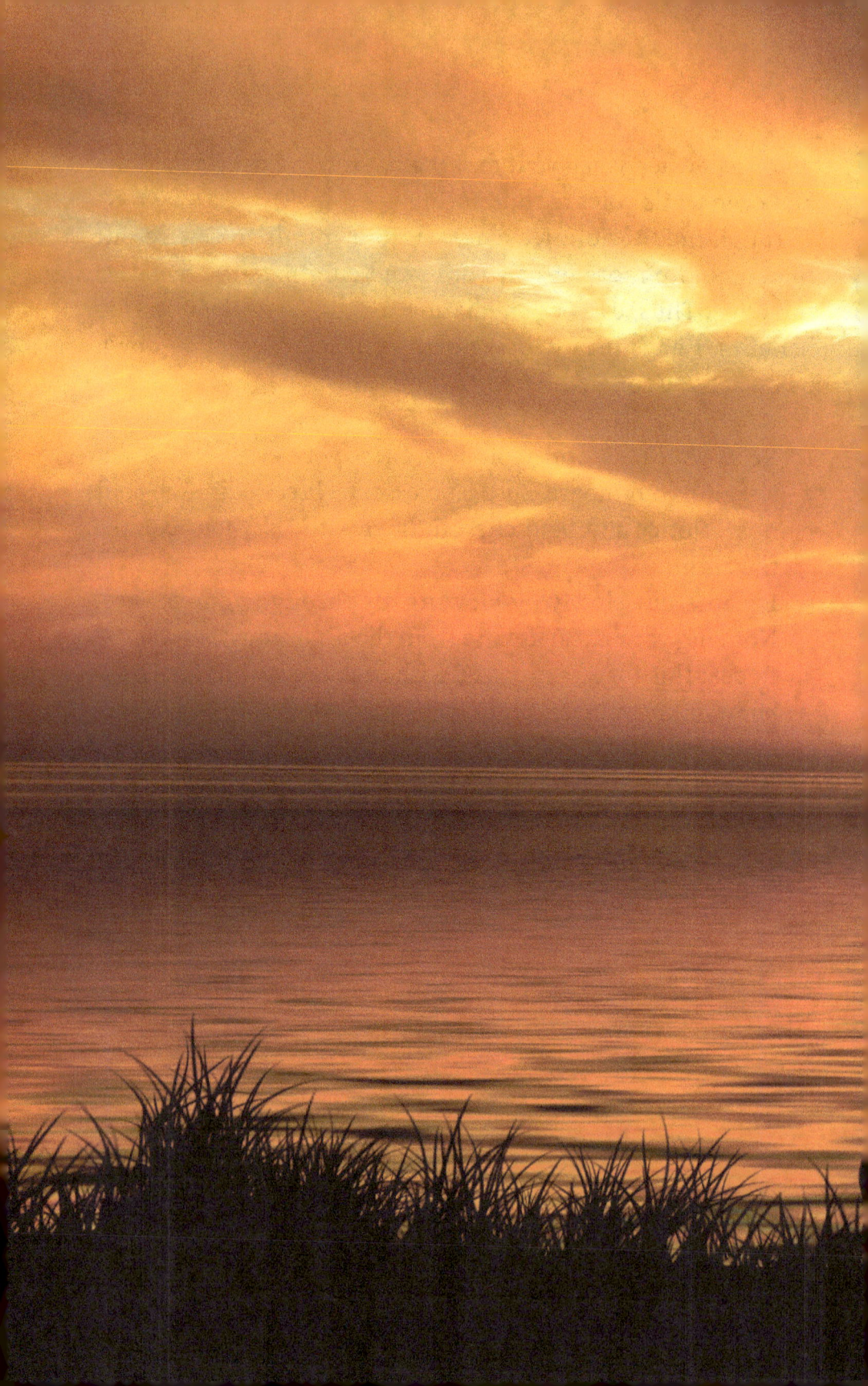

MONDAY

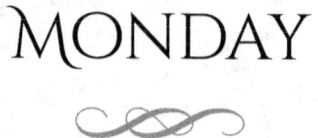

Morning Session

Find a quote, lyric, a picture, or something you have heard and stick it underneath. This is what you are going to start your day with! Make it funny or positive. Just as long as it makes you feel good. It is your dandelion in the concreate for the day!

Now write 5 goals that you want to achieve today. Remember you can make them small, medium or big, but make them achievable! Do not write things that you will not be able to achieve and whatever you cannot complete today does not roll over to tomorrow.

1. _____

_____

2. _____

_____

3. _____

_____

4. _____

_____

5. _____

_____

Evening Session

Reflect on your day and now write 5 things or people that you are grateful for! Be Specific about your day. Remember you can be grateful for people, yourself or objects.

1. _____

_____

2. _____

_____

3. _____

_____

4. _____

_____

5. _____

_____

Has it been a hard day? This is where you write 5 things or people you want to forgive. Again, do not forget to be specific about the day! And remember you can include yourself, people or objects.

1. _____

   _____

2. _____

   _____

3. _____

   _____

4. _____

   _____

5. _____

   _____

Reflection Space

This is your space! This is where you can make a few notes, you can do a spider diagram, you can doodle, or you can simply write down how you feel. If you are going to write down how you feel, remember to not rant and whine about your day, but to think of about, what you have learnt from the day and how you could improve for the next day. Ranting and moaning about the day will only create negative emotions and leave you feeling down. Keep it positive!

TUESDAY

Morning Session

Find a quote, lyric, a picture, or something you have heard and stick it underneath. This is what you are going to start your day with! Make it funny or positive. Just as long as it makes you feel good. It is your dandelion in the concrete for the day!

Now write 5 goals that you want to achieve today. Remember you can make them small, medium or big, but make them achievable! Do not write things that you will not be able to achieve and whatever you cannot complete today does not roll over to tomorrow.

1. _____

   _____

2. _____

   _____

3. _____

   _____

4. _____

   _____

5. _____

   _____

Evening Session

Reflect on your day and now write 5 things or people that you are grateful for! Be Specific about your day. Remember you can be grateful for people, yourself or objects.

1. _____

   _____

2. _____

   _____

3. _____

   _____

4. _____

   _____

5. _____

   _____

Has it been a hard day? This is where you write 5 things or people you want to forgive. Again, do not forget to be specific about the day! And remember you can include yourself, people or objects.

1. _____

   _____

2. _____

   _____

3. _____

   _____

4. _____

   _____

5. _____

   _____

Reflection Space

This is your space! This is where you can make a few notes, you can do a spider diagram, you can doodle, or you can simply write down how you feel. If you are going to write down how you feel, remember to not rant and whine about your day, but to think of about, what you have learnt from the day and how you could improve for the next day. Ranting and moaning about the day will only create negative emotions and leave you feeling down. Keep it positive!

WEDNESDAY

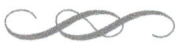

Morning Session

Find a quote, lyric, a picture, or something you have heard and stick it underneath. This is what you are going to start your day with! Make it funny or positive. Just as long as it makes you feel good. It is your dandelion in the concrete for the day!

Now write 5 goals that you want to achieve today. Remember you can make them small, medium or big, but make them achievable! Do not write things that you will not be able to achieve and whatever you cannot complete today does not roll over to tomorrow.

1. _____

   _____

2. _____

   _____

3. _____

   _____

4. _____

   _____

5. _____

   _____

Evening Session

Reflect on your day and now write 5 things or people that you are grateful for! Be Specific about your day. Remember you can be grateful for people, yourself or objects.

1. _____

_____

2. _____

_____

3. _____

_____

4. _____

_____

5. _____

_____

Has it been a hard day? This is where you write 5 things or people you want to forgive. Again, do not forget to be specific about the day! And remember you can include yourself, people or objects.

1. _____

_____

2. _____

_____

3. _____

_____

4. _____

_____

5. _____

_____

Reflection Space

This is your space! This is where you can make a few notes, you can do a spider diagram, you can doodle, or you can simply write down how you feel. If you are going to write down how you feel, remember to not rant and whine about your day, but to think of about, what you have learnt from the day and how you could improve for the next day. Ranting and moaning about the day will only create negative emotions and leave you feeling down. Keep it positive!

THURSDAY

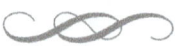

Morning Session

Find a quote, lyric, a picture, or something you have heard and stick it underneath. This is what you are going to start your day with! Make it funny or positive. Just as long as it makes you feel good. It is your dandelion in the concreate for the day!

Now write 5 goals that you want to achieve today. Remember you can make them small, medium or big, but make them achievable! Do not write things that you will not be able to achieve and whatever you cannot complete today does not roll over to tomorrow.

1. _____

   _____

2. _____

   _____

3. _____

   _____

4. _____

   _____

5. _____

   _____

Evening Session

Reflect on your day and now write 5 things or people that you are grateful for! Be Specific about your day. Remember you can be grateful for people, yourself or objects.

1. _____

   _____

2. _____

   _____

3. _____

   _____

4. _____

   _____

5. _____

   _____

Has it been a hard day? This is where you write 5 things or people you want to forgive. Again, do not forget to be specific about the day! And remember you can include yourself, people or objects.

1. _____

   _____

2. _____

   _____

3. _____

   _____

4. _____

   _____

5. _____

   _____

Reflection Space

This is your space! This is where you can make a few notes, you can do a spider diagram, you can doodle, or you can simply write down how you feel. If you are going to write down how you feel, remember to not rant and whine about your day, but to think of about, what you have learnt from the day and how you could improve for the next day. Ranting and moaning about the day will only create negative emotions and leave you feeling down. Keep it positive!

FRIDAY

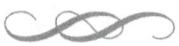

Morning Session

Find a quote, lyric, a picture, or something you have heard and stick it underneath. This is what you are going to start your day with! Make it funny or positive. Just as long as it makes you feel good. It is your dandelion in the concreate for the day!

Now write 5 goals that you want to achieve today. Remember you can make them small, medium or big, but make them achievable! Do not write things that you will not be able to achieve and whatever you cannot complete today does not roll over to tomorrow.

1. _____

   _____

2. _____

   _____

3. _____

   _____

4. _____

   _____

5. _____

   _____

Evening Session

Reflect on your day and now write 5 things or people that you are grateful for! Be Specific about your day. Remember you can be grateful for people, yourself or objects.

1. _____

   _____

2. _____

   _____

3. _____

   _____

4. _____

   _____

5. _____

   _____

Has it been a hard day? This is where you write 5 things or people you want to forgive. Again, do not forget to be specific about the day! And remember you can include yourself, people or objects.

1. _____

   _____

2. _____

   _____

3. _____

   _____

4. _____

   _____

5. _____

   _____

Reflection Space

This is your space! This is where you can make a few notes, you can do a spider diagram, you can doodle, or you can simply write down how you feel. If you are going to write down how you feel, remember to not rant and whine about your day, but to think of about, what you have learnt from the day and how you could improve for the next day. Ranting and moaning about the day will only create negative emotions and leave you feeling down. Keep it positive!

SATURDAY

Morning Session

Find a quote, lyric, a picture, or something you have heard and stick it underneath. This is what you are going to start your day with! Make it funny or positive. Just as long as it makes you feel good. It is your dandelion in the concreate for the day!

Now write 5 goals that you want to achieve today. Remember you can make them small, medium or big, but make them achievable! Do not write things that you will not be able to achieve and whatever you cannot complete today does not roll over to tomorrow.

1. _____

   _____

2. _____

   _____

3. _____

   _____

4. _____

   _____

5. _____

   _____

Evening Session

Reflect on your day and now write 5 things or people that you are grateful for! Be Specific about your day. Remember you can be grateful for people, yourself or objects.

1. _____

_____

2. _____

_____

3. _____

_____

4. _____

_____

5. _____

_____

Has it been a hard day? This is where you write 5 things or people you want to forgive. Again, do not forget to be specific about the day! And remember you can include yourself, people or objects.

1. _____

_____

2. _____

_____

3. _____

_____

4. _____

_____

5. _____

_____

Reflection Space

This is your space! This is where you can make a few notes, you can do a spider diagram, you can doodle, or you can simply write down how you feel. If you are going to write down how you feel, remember to not rant and whine about your day, but to think of about, what you have learnt from the day and how you could improve for the next day. Ranting and moaning about the day will only create negative emotions and leave you feeling down. Keep it positive!

SUNDAY

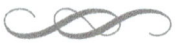

Morning Session

Find a quote, lyric, a picture, or something you have heard and stick it underneath. This is what you are going to start your day with! Make it funny or positive. Just as long as it makes you feel good. It is your dandelion in the concreate for the day!

Now write 5 goals that you want to achieve today. Remember you can make them small, medium or big, but make them achievable! Do not write things that you will not be able to achieve and whatever you cannot complete today does not roll over to tomorrow.

1. _____

   _____

2. _____

   _____

3. _____

   _____

4. _____

   _____

5. _____

   _____

Evening Session

Reflect on your day and now write 5 things or people that you are grateful for! Be Specific about your day. Remember you can be grateful for people, yourself or objects.

1. _____

   _____

2. _____

   _____

3. _____

   _____

4. _____

   _____

5. _____

   _____

Has it been a hard day? This is where you write 5 things or people you want to forgive. Again, do not forget to be specific about the day! And remember you can include yourself, people or objects.

1. _____

   _____

2. _____

   _____

3. _____

   _____

4. _____

   _____

5. _____

   _____

Reflection Space

This is your space! This is where you can make a few notes, you can do a spider diagram, you can doodle, or you can simply write down how you feel. If you are going to write down how you feel, remember to not rant and whine about your day, but to think of about, what you have learnt from the day and how you could improve for the next day. Ranting and moaning about the day will only create negative emotions and leave you feeling down. Keep it positive!

EATING HEALTHY

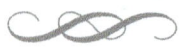

Our brains are constantly working and for our brains to work, like any other organ, require different amounts vitamins, minerals and carbohydrates to function and what you eat can directly affect your mental health. In recent years, the relationship between diet and mental health have gained considerable interest and has shown that feeding the brain with a diet that provides adequate amounts of complex carbohydrates, essential fats, amino acids, vitamins, minerals and water can support healthy neurotransmitter activities. This can then protect the brain from the effects of oxidants, which have been shown negatively to impact mood and mental health.

Latest research has shown that the Mediterranean diet and the Japanese diet compared to the Western diet is a 25% risk of depression compared to 35% with those on a western diet. This is because the studies have shown that the Mediterranean diet and the Japanese diet tends to be high in vegetables, fruits, unprocessed grains and fish and seafood and contains little lean meat and dairy. The diets also contain extraordinarily little processed and refined foods and sugars which are very much prominent in the Western diet.

It is important to mention here that mood can also affect our food choices. When we are feeling low, we are conditioned to reach out for a high processed carbohydrate food diet which could then increase our risk of depression and anxiety, therefore entering a cycle with our diet and our mood.

Our moods can also be affected by drinking too much alcohol. Alcohol is known to have a depressive factor, and this can lead to a deterioration in mood and can have effect on your sleep patterns, which can then lead to reduce energy levels. Alcohol then depresses the central nervous system, and this can also make your moods fluctuate. Although alcohol can be used to numb our emotions at times, it can do so only for a short period of time before sending us down crashing in a sea of emotions which we may find overwhelming.

Having a balanced diet refers to eating a variety of food with the right proportions whilst thinking about the quality of food that you eat and the kinds of food you eat, for example, how many calories it may contain? Whether it is processed or not and the timing you may eat your food.

The best way to do this is to start paying attention to how eating different foods makes you feel, not just in the moment, but the next day. Try eating a "clean" diet for two to three weeks, that means cutting out all processed foods and sugar and see how you feel. Then slowly introduce foods back into your diet, one by one, and see how you feel. This way you will be a better understanding of what foods are better suited to you and your body.

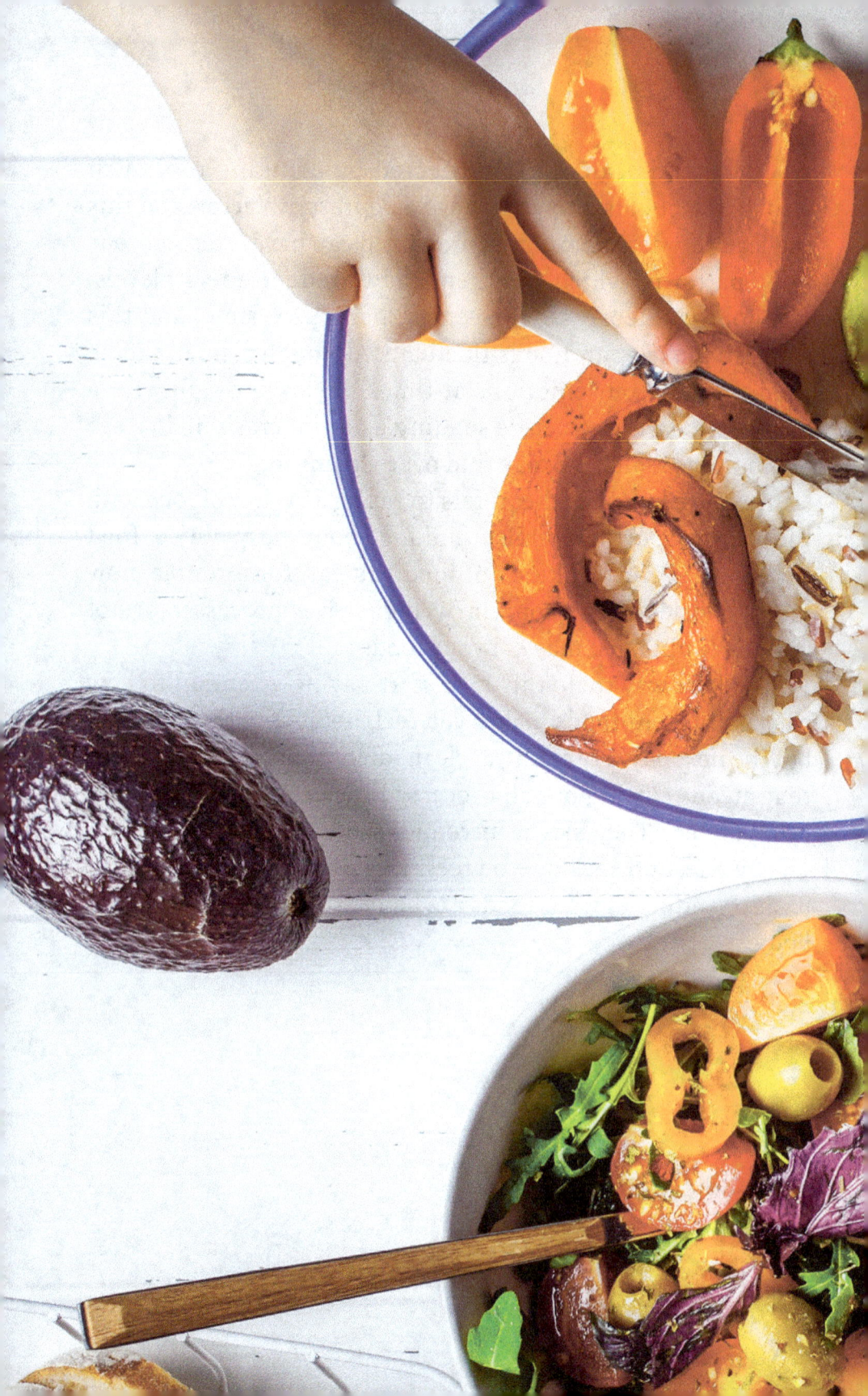

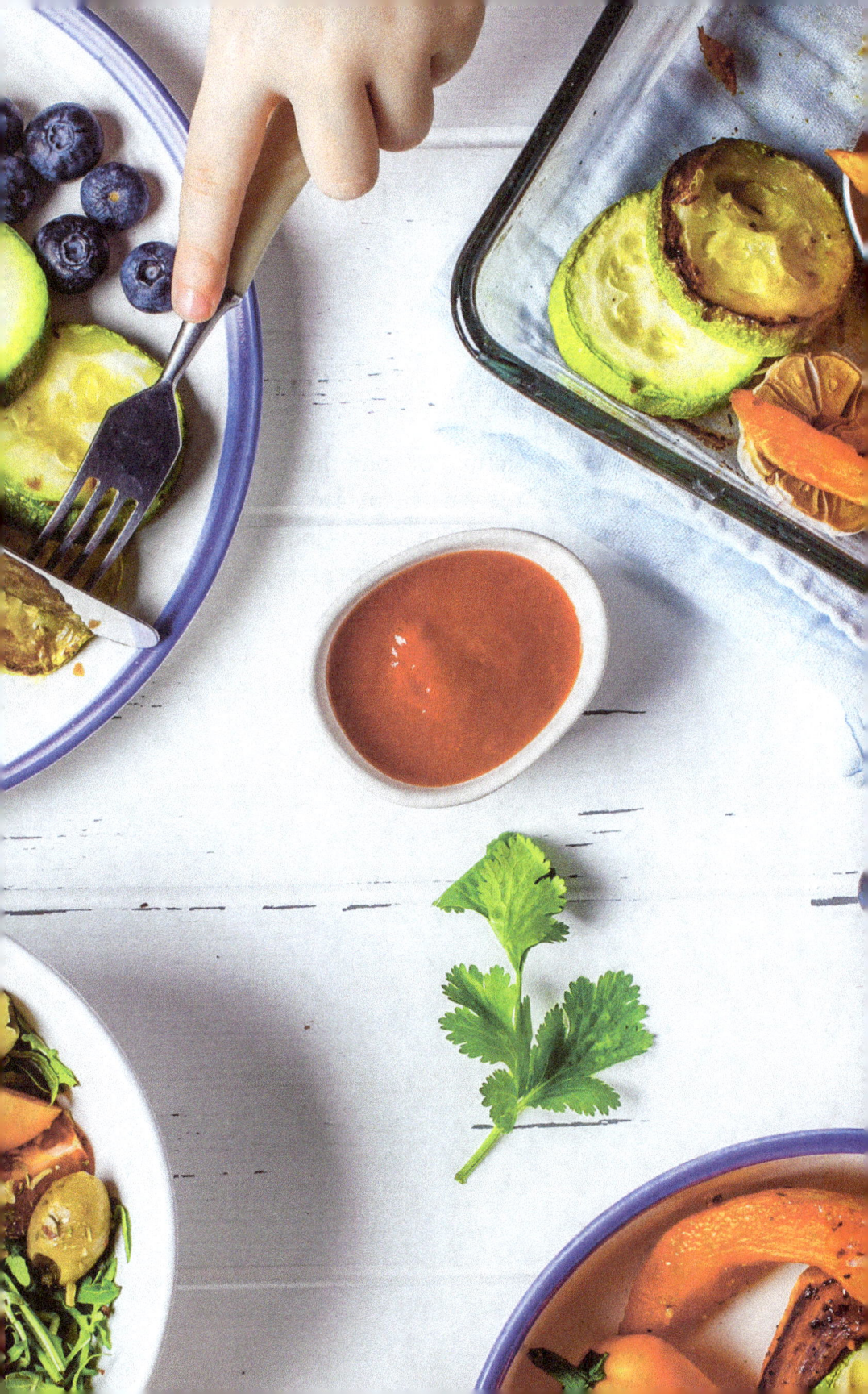

MONDAY

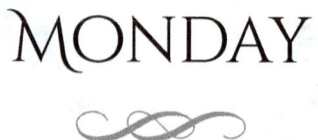

Morning Session

Find a quote, lyric, a picture, or something you have heard and stick it underneath. This is what you are going to start your day with! Make it funny or positive. Just as long as it makes you feel good. It is your dandelion in the concrete for the day!

Now write 5 goals that you want to achieve today. Remember you can make them small, medium or big, but make them achievable! Do not write things that you will not be able to achieve and whatever you cannot complete today does not roll over to tomorrow.

1. _____

   _____

2. _____

   _____

3. _____

   _____

4. _____

   _____

5. _____

   _____

Evening Session

Reflect on your day and now write 5 things or people that you are grateful for! Be Specific about your day. Remember you can be grateful for people, yourself or objects.

1. _____

_____

2. _____

_____

3. _____

_____

4. _____

_____

5. _____

_____

Has it been a hard day? This is where you write 5 things or people you want to forgive. Again, do not forget to be specific about the day! And remember you can include yourself, people or objects.

1. _____
   _____

2. _____
   _____

3. _____
   _____

4. _____
   _____

5. _____
   _____

Reflection Space

This is your space! This is where you can make a few notes, you can do a spider diagram, you can doodle, or you can simply write down how you feel. If you are going to write down how you feel, remember to not rant and whine about your day, but to think of about, what you have learnt from the day and how you could improve for the next day. Ranting and moaning about the day will only create negative emotions and leave you feeling down. Keep it positive!

TUESDAY

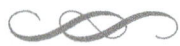

Morning Session

Find a quote, lyric, a picture, or something you have heard and stick it underneath. This is what you are going to start your day with! Make it funny or positive. Just as long as it makes you feel good. It is your dandelion in the concreate for the day!

Now write 5 goals that you want to achieve today. Remember you can make them small, medium or big, but make them achievable! Do not write things that you will not be able to achieve and whatever you cannot complete today does not roll over to tomorrow.

1. _____

   _____

2. _____

   _____

3. _____

   _____

4. _____

   _____

5. _____

   _____

   _____

Evening Session

Reflect on your day and now write 5 things or people that you are grateful for! Be Specific about your day. Remember you can be grateful for people, yourself or objects.

1. _____

   _____

2. _____

   _____

3. _____

   _____

4. _____

   _____

5. _____

   _____

   _____

Has it been a hard day? This is where you write 5 things or people you want to forgive. Again, do not forget to be specific about the day! And remember you can include yourself, people or objects.

1. _____

   _____

2. _____

   _____

3. _____

   _____

4. _____

   _____

5. _____

   _____

   _____

Reflection Space

This is your space! This is where you can make a few notes, you can do a spider diagram, you can doodle, or you can simply write down how you feel. If you are going to write down how you feel, remember to not rant and whine about your day, but to think of about, what you have learnt from the day and how you could improve for the next day. Ranting and moaning about the day will only create negative emotions and leave you feeling down. Keep it positive!

WEDNESDAY

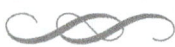

Morning Session

Find a quote, lyric, a picture, or something you have heard and stick it underneath. This is what you are going to start your day with! Make it funny or positive. Just as long as it makes you feel good. It is your dandelion in the concreate for the day!

Now write 5 goals that you want to achieve today. Remember you can make them small, medium or big, but make them achievable! Do not write things that you will not be able to achieve and whatever you cannot complete today does not roll over to tomorrow.

1. _____

   _____

2. _____

   _____

3. _____

   _____

4. _____

   _____

5. _____

   _____

   _____

Evening Session

Reflect on your day and now write 5 things or people that you are grateful for! Be Specific about your day. Remember you can be grateful for people, yourself or objects.

1. _____

   _____

2. _____

   _____

3. _____

   _____

4. _____

   _____

5. _____

   _____

Has it been a hard day? This is where you write 5 things or people you want to forgive. Again, do not forget to be specific about the day! And remember you can include yourself, people or objects.

1. _____

   _____

2. _____

   _____

3. _____

   _____

4. _____

   _____

5. _____

   _____

Reflection Space

This is your space! This is where you can make a few notes, you can do a spider diagram, you can doodle, or you can simply write down how you feel. If you are going to write down how you feel, remember to not rant and whine about your day, but to think of about, what you have learnt from the day and how you could improve for the next day. Ranting and moaning about the day will only create negative emotions and leave you feeling down. Keep it positive!

THURSDAY

Morning Session

Find a quote, lyric, a picture, or something you have heard and stick it underneath. This is what you are going to start your day with! Make it funny or positive. Just as long as it makes you feel good. It is your dandelion in the concrete for the day!

Now write 5 goals that you want to achieve today. Remember you can make them small, medium or big, but make them achievable! Do not write things that you will not be able to achieve and whatever you cannot complete today does not roll over to tomorrow.

1. _____

   _____

2. _____

   _____

3. _____

   _____

4. _____

   _____

5. _____

   _____

Evening Session

Reflect on your day and now write 5 things or people that you are grateful for! Be Specific about your day. Remember you can be grateful for people, yourself or objects.

1. _____

_____

2. _____

_____

3. _____

_____

4. _____

_____

5. _____

_____

Has it been a hard day? This is where you write 5 things or people you want to forgive. Again, do not forget to be specific about the day! And remember you can include yourself, people or objects.

1. _____

   _____

2. _____

   _____

3. _____

   _____

4. _____

   _____

5. _____

   _____

Reflection Space

This is your space! This is where you can make a few notes, you can do a spider diagram, you can doodle, or you can simply write down how you feel. If you are going to write down how you feel, remember to not rant and whine about your day, but to think of about, what you have learnt from the day and how you could improve for the next day. Ranting and moaning about the day will only create negative emotions and leave you feeling down. Keep it positive!

FRIDAY

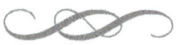

Morning Session

Find a quote, lyric, a picture, or something you have heard and stick it underneath. This is what you are going to start your day with! Make it funny or positive. Just as long as it makes you feel good. It is your dandelion in the concreate for the day!

Now write 5 goals that you want to achieve today. Remember you can make them small, medium or big, but make them achievable! Do not write things that you will not be able to achieve and whatever you cannot complete today does not roll over to tomorrow.

1. _____

   _____

2. _____

   _____

3. _____

   _____

4. _____

   _____

5. _____

   _____

Evening Session

Reflect on your day and now write 5 things or people that you are grateful for! Be Specific about your day. Remember you can be grateful for people, yourself or objects.

1. _____

   _____

2. _____

   _____

3. _____

   _____

4. _____

   _____

5. _____

   _____

Has it been a hard day? This is where you write 5 things or people you want to forgive. Again, do not forget to be specific about the day! And remember you can include yourself, people or objects.

1. _____

   _____

2. _____

   _____

3. _____

   _____

4. _____

   _____

5. _____

   _____

Reflection Space

This is your space! This is where you can make a few notes, you can do a spider diagram, you can doodle, or you can simply write down how you feel. If you are going to write down how you feel, remember to not rant and whine about your day, but to think of about, what you have learnt from the day and how you could improve for the next day. Ranting and moaning about the day will only create negative emotions and leave you feeling down. Keep it positive!

SATURDAY

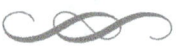

Morning Session

Find a quote, lyric, a picture, or something you have heard and stick it underneath. This is what you are going to start your day with! Make it funny or positive. Just as long as it makes you feel good. It is your dandelion in the concreate for the day!

Now write 5 goals that you want to achieve today. Remember you can make them small, medium or big, but make them achievable! Do not write things that you will not be able to achieve and whatever you cannot complete today does not roll over to tomorrow.

1. _____

   _____

2. _____

   _____

3. _____

   _____

4. _____

   _____

5. _____

   _____

Evening Session

Reflect on your day and now write 5 things or people that you are grateful for! Be Specific about your day. Remember you can be grateful for people, yourself or objects.

1. _____

   _____

2. _____

   _____

3. _____

   _____

4. _____

   _____

5. _____

   _____

Has it been a hard day? This is where you write 5 things or people you want to forgive. Again, do not forget to be specific about the day! And remember you can include yourself, people or objects.

1. _____

   _____

2. _____

   _____

3. _____

   _____

4. _____

   _____

5. _____

   _____

Reflection Space

This is your space! This is where you can make a few notes, you can do a spider diagram, you can doodle, or you can simply write down how you feel. If you are going to write down how you feel, remember to not rant and whine about your day, but to think of about, what you have learnt from the day and how you could improve for the next day. Ranting and moaning about the day will only create negative emotions and leave you feeling down. Keep it positive!

SUNDAY

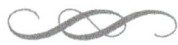

Morning Session

Find a quote, lyric, a picture, or something you have heard and stick it underneath. This is what you are going to start your day with! Make it funny or positive. Just as long as it makes you feel good. It is your dandelion in the concreate for the day!

Now write 5 goals that you want to achieve today. Remember you can make them small, medium or big, but make them achievable! Do not write things that you will not be able to achieve and whatever you cannot complete today does not roll over to tomorrow.

1. _____

   _____

2. _____

   _____

3. _____

   _____

4. _____

   _____

5. _____

   _____

Evening Session

Reflect on your day and now write 5 things or people that you are grateful for! Be Specific about your day. Remember you can be grateful for people, yourself or objects.

1. _____

   _____

2. _____

   _____

3. _____

   _____

4. _____

   _____

5. _____

   _____

Has it been a hard day? This is where you write 5 things or people you want to forgive. Again, do not forget to be specific about the day! And remember you can include yourself, people or objects.

1. _____

   _____

2. _____

   _____

3. _____

   _____

4. _____

   _____

5. _____

   _____

Reflection Space

This is your space! This is where you can make a few notes, you can do a spider diagram, you can doodle, or you can simply write down how you feel. If you are going to write down how you feel, remember to not rant and whine about your day, but to think of about, what you have learnt from the day and how you could improve for the next day. Ranting and moaning about the day will only create negative emotions and leave you feeling down. Keep it positive!

IMPROVING YOUR SELF ESTEEM

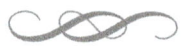

Self esteem is our own evaluation of what we think of ourselves and can often include other people's perception of you. When we are feeling good, we tend to feel positive about ourselves and life in general. Therefore, we are better equipped to deal with life's ups and downs and are more resilient. When we feel low about ourselves, this can affect, not only the way we think about our ourselves, but make us more critical of others and the world around us. It also makes it a lot harder to bounce back from challenges and setbacks, which can then lead to bouts of depression and anxiety.

There are multiple reasons why a person's self esteem could be low. Sometimes it may have started as early as childhood, where you felt that you did not live up to an expectation that was set whether it was in school, by friends, or home. Or it could have started in later life because of a relationship, or work where you might have felt vulnerable or felt insecure. The positive news is that you have the power to change your self-esteem, if you think your self-esteem is low.

The most important thing to do to help improve your self esteem is to be kind to yourself. Start using kinder words to describe yourself and be positive about the things that you can do. Start loving who you are and enjoy being around yourself. Do not compare yourself with others and look at what others have. Remember that you are an individual and things will come to you when the universe is ready to bring them to you and you do not know what paths other people have walked to get what they have. Start to identify any negative thoughts and beliefs that you might have and turn them around. At first, they will not feel comfortable to you because you will not be used to saying nice things to yourself but gradually you will learn to love saying great things about yourself.

To have a good self-esteem, you need good positive people in your life and around your life. Make a vow to yourself to surround yourself with positive people who will influence you and who will lift you up. You do not want people who will put you down or who will constantly break your spirit even if they are telling you that they are doing it for your own good because the chances are, they are doing it to bring themselves up and to keep you in a position where they can feel good about themselves.

Be the person you want to be and not the person you feel is expected of you and be proud of who you. Give yourself that permission and allow yourself to be free of all the social stipulations that may be put on you.

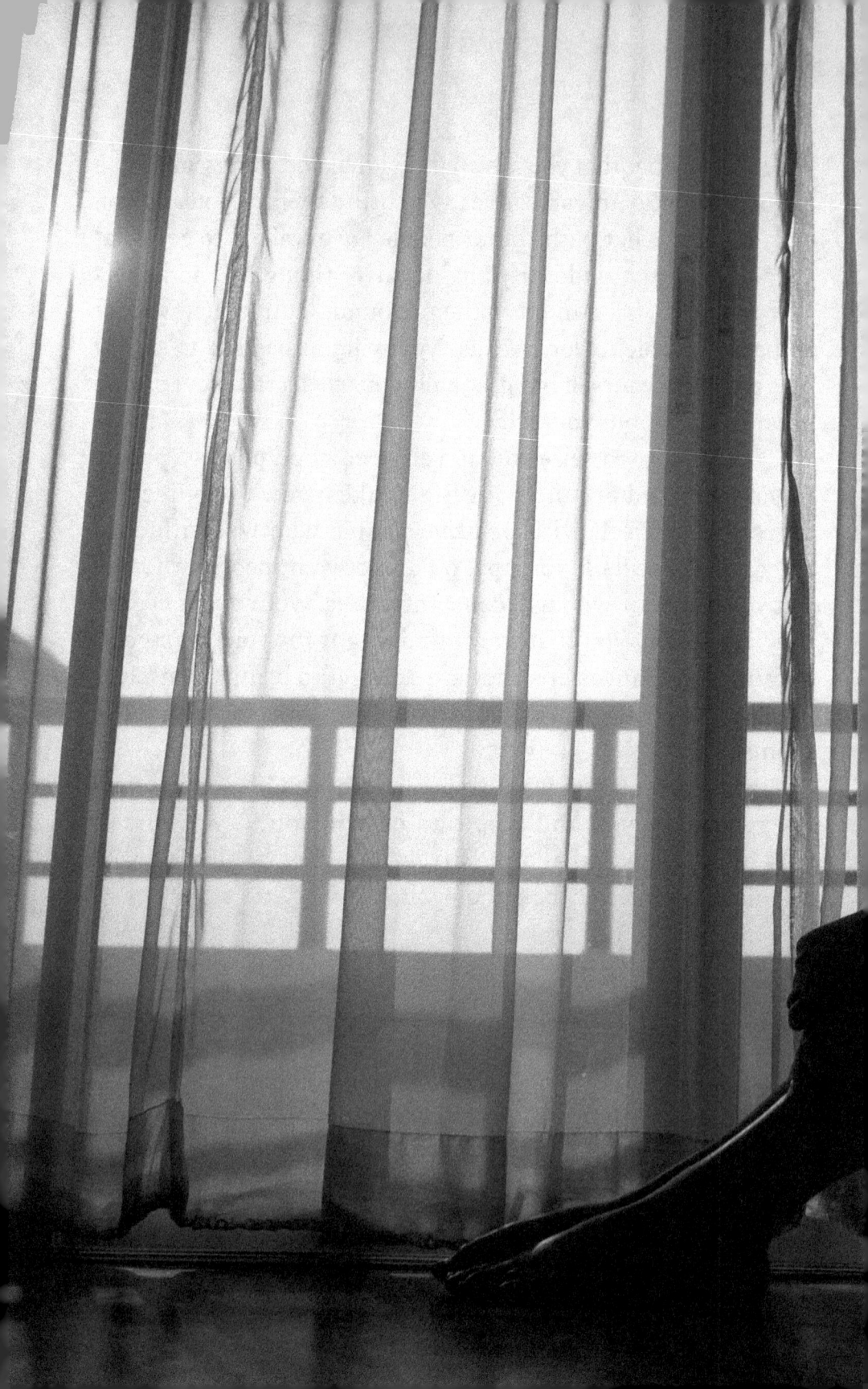

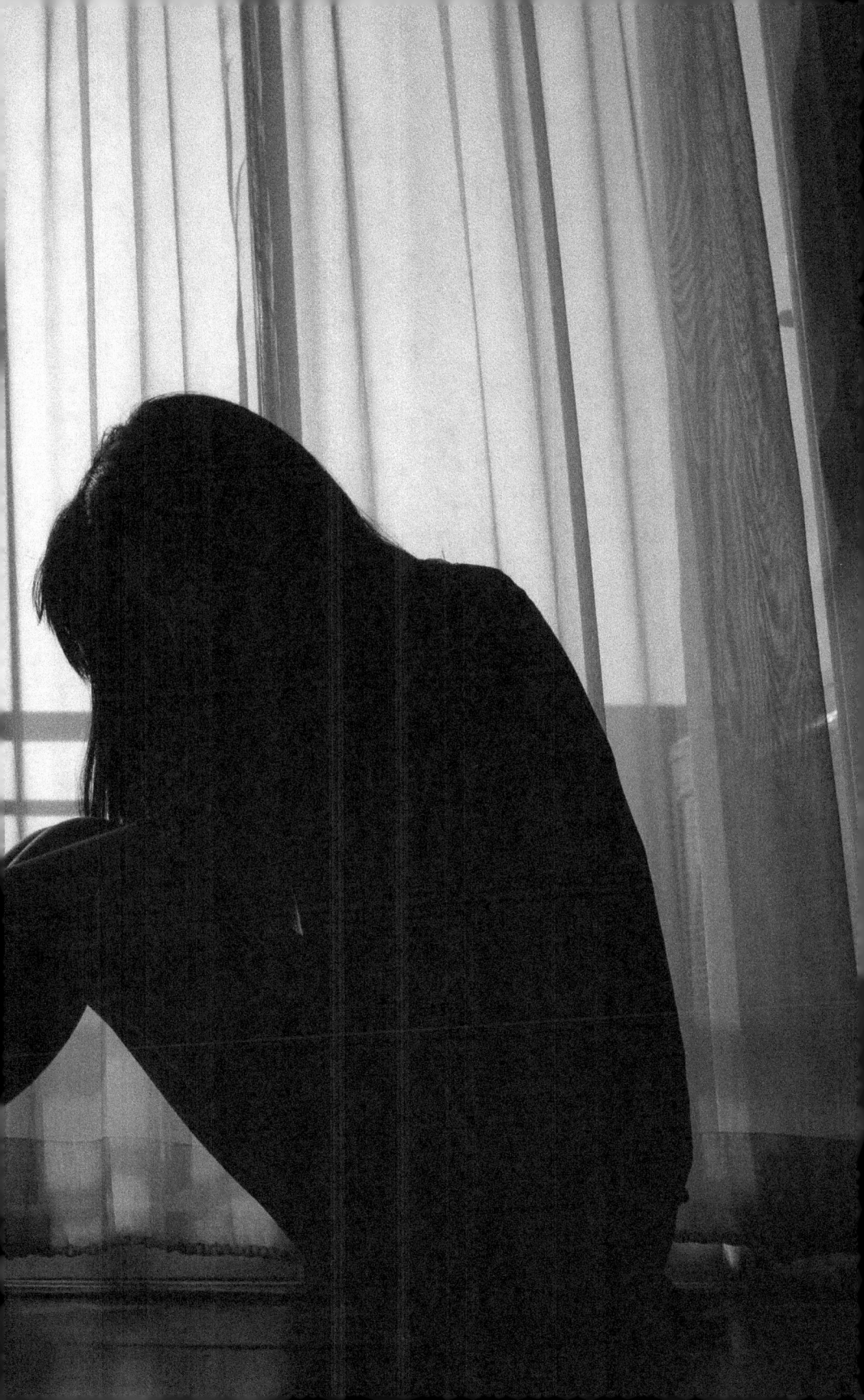

MONDAY

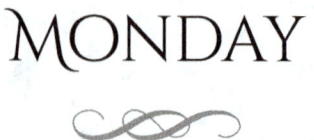

Morning Session

Find a quote, lyric, a picture, or something you have heard and stick it underneath. This is what you are going to start your day with! Make it funny or positive. Just as long as it makes you feel good. It is your dandelion in the concreate for the day!

Now write 5 goals that you want to achieve today. Remember you can make them small, medium or big, but make them achievable! Do not write things that you will not be able to achieve and whatever you cannot complete today does not roll over to tomorrow.

1. _____

   _____

2. _____

   _____

3. _____

   _____

4. _____

   _____

5. _____

   _____

   _____

Evening Session

Reflect on your day and now write 5 things or people that you are grateful for! Be Specific about your day. Remember you can be grateful for people, yourself or objects.

1. _____

   _____

2. _____

   _____

3. _____

   _____

4. _____

   _____

5. _____

   _____

Has it been a hard day? This is where you write 5 things or people you want to forgive. Again, do not forget to be specific about the day! And remember you can include yourself, people or objects.

1. _____

   _____

2. _____

   _____

3. _____

   _____

4. _____

   _____

5. _____

   _____

   _____

Reflection Space

This is your space! This is where you can make a few notes, you can do a spider diagram, you can doodle, or you can simply write down how you feel. If you are going to write down how you feel, remember to not rant and whine about your day, but to think of about, what you have learnt from the day and how you could improve for the next day. Ranting and moaning about the day will only create negative emotions and leave you feeling down. Keep it positive!

TUESDAY

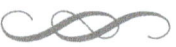

Morning Session

Find a quote, lyric, a picture, or something you have heard and stick it underneath. This is what you are going to start your day with! Make it funny or positive. Just as long as it makes you feel good. It is your dandelion in the concreate for the day!

Now write 5 goals that you want to achieve today. Remember you can make them small, medium or big, but make them achievable! Do not write things that you will not be able to achieve and whatever you cannot complete today does not roll over to tomorrow.

1. _____

   _____

2. _____

   _____

3. _____

   _____

4. _____

   _____

5. _____

   _____

Evening Session

Reflect on your day and now write 5 things or people that you are grateful for! Be Specific about your day. Remember you can be grateful for people, yourself or objects.

1. _____

   _____

2. _____

   _____

3. _____

   _____

4. _____

   _____

5. _____

   _____

Has it been a hard day? This is where you write 5 things or people you want to forgive. Again, do not forget to be specific about the day! And remember you can include yourself, people or objects.

1. _____

   _____

2. _____

   _____

3. _____

   _____

4. _____

   _____

5. _____

   _____

Reflection Space

This is your space! This is where you can make a few notes, you can do a spider diagram, you can doodle, or you can simply write down how you feel. If you are going to write down how you feel, remember to not rant and whine about your day, but to think of about, what you have learnt from the day and how you could improve for the next day. Ranting and moaning about the day will only create negative emotions and leave you feeling down. Keep it positive!

WEDNESDAY

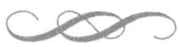

Morning Session

Find a quote, lyric, a picture, or something you have heard and stick it underneath. This is what you are going to start your day with! Make it funny or positive. Just as long as it makes you feel good. It is your dandelion in the concreate for the day!

Now write 5 goals that you want to achieve today. Remember you can make them small, medium or big, but make them achievable! Do not write things that you will not be able to achieve and whatever you cannot complete today does not roll over to tomorrow.

1. _____

_____

2. _____

_____

3. _____

_____

4. _____

_____

5. _____

_____

Evening Session

Reflect on your day and now write 5 things or people that you are grateful for! Be Specific about your day. Remember you can be grateful for people, yourself or objects.

1. _____

   _____

2. _____

   _____

3. _____

   _____

4. _____

   _____

5. _____

   _____

Has it been a hard day? This is where you write 5 things or people you want to forgive. Again, do not forget to be specific about the day! And remember you can include yourself, people or objects.

1. _____

   _____

2. _____

   _____

3. _____

   _____

4. _____

   _____

5. _____

   _____

Reflection Space

This is your space! This is where you can make a few notes, you can do a spider diagram, you can doodle, or you can simply write down how you feel. If you are going to write down how you feel, remember to not rant and whine about your day, but to think of about, what you have learnt from the day and how you could improve for the next day. Ranting and moaning about the day will only create negative emotions and leave you feeling down. Keep it positive!

THURSDAY

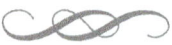

Morning Session

Find a quote, lyric, a picture, or something you have heard and stick it underneath. This is what you are going to start your day with! Make it funny or positive. Just as long as it makes you feel good. It is your dandelion in the concreate for the day!

Now write 5 goals that you want to achieve today. Remember you can make them small, medium or big, but make them achievable! Do not write things that you will not be able to achieve and whatever you cannot complete today does not roll over to tomorrow.

1. _____

   _____

2. _____

   _____

3. _____

   _____

4. _____

   _____

5. _____

   _____

Evening Session

Reflect on your day and now write 5 things or people that you are grateful for! Be Specific about your day. Remember you can be grateful for people, yourself or objects.

1. _____

_____

2. _____

_____

3. _____

_____

4. _____

_____

5. _____

_____

Has it been a hard day? This is where you write 5 things or people you want to forgive. Again, do not forget to be specific about the day! And remember you can include yourself, people or objects.

1. _____

   _____

2. _____

   _____

3. _____

   _____

4. _____

   _____

5. _____

   _____

Reflection Space

This is your space! This is where you can make a few notes, you can do a spider diagram, you can doodle, or you can simply write down how you feel. If you are going to write down how you feel, remember to not rant and whine about your day, but to think of about, what you have learnt from the day and how you could improve for the next day. Ranting and moaning about the day will only create negative emotions and leave you feeling down. Keep it positive!

FRIDAY

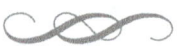

Morning Session

Find a quote, lyric, a picture, or something you have heard and stick it underneath. This is what you are going to start your day with! Make it funny or positive. Just as long as it makes you feel good. It is your dandelion in the concrete for the day!

Now write 5 goals that you want to achieve today. Remember you can make them small, medium or big, but make them achievable! Do not write things that you will not be able to achieve and whatever you cannot complete today does not roll over to tomorrow.

1. _____

   _____

2. _____

   _____

3. _____

   _____

4. _____

   _____

5. _____

   _____

Evening Session

Reflect on your day and now write 5 things or people that you are grateful for! Be Specific about your day. Remember you can be grateful for people, yourself or objects.

1. _____

_____

2. _____

_____

3. _____

_____

4. _____

_____

5. _____

_____

Has it been a hard day? This is where you write 5 things or people you want to forgive. Again, do not forget to be specific about the day! And remember you can include yourself, people or objects.

1. _____

   _____

2. _____

   _____

3. _____

   _____

4. _____

   _____

5. _____

   _____

Reflection Space

This is your space! This is where you can make a few notes, you can do a spider diagram, you can doodle, or you can simply write down how you feel. If you are going to write down how you feel, remember to not rant and whine about your day, but to think of about, what you have learnt from the day and how you could improve for the next day. Ranting and moaning about the day will only create negative emotions and leave you feeling down. Keep it positive!

SATURDAY

Morning Session

Find a quote, lyric, a picture, or something you have heard and stick it underneath. This is what you are going to start your day with! Make it funny or positive. Just as long as it makes you feel good. It is your dandelion in the concreate for the day!

Now write 5 goals that you want to achieve today. Remember you can make them small, medium or big, but make them achievable! Do not write things that you will not be able to achieve and whatever you cannot complete today does not roll over to tomorrow.

1. _____

   _____

2. _____

   _____

3. _____

   _____

4. _____

   _____

5. _____

   _____

Evening Session

Reflect on your day and now write 5 things or people that you are grateful for! Be Specific about your day. Remember you can be grateful for people, yourself or objects.

1. _____

_____

2. _____

_____

3. _____

_____

4. _____

_____

5. _____

_____

Has it been a hard day? This is where you write 5 things or people you want to forgive. Again, do not forget to be specific about the day! And remember you can include yourself, people or objects.

1. _____

   _____

2. _____

   _____

3. _____

   _____

4. _____

   _____

5. _____

   _____

Reflection Space

This is your space! This is where you can make a few notes, you can do a spider diagram, you can doodle, or you can simply write down how you feel. If you are going to write down how you feel, remember to not rant and whine about your day, but to think of about, what you have learnt from the day and how you could improve for the next day. Ranting and moaning about the day will only create negative emotions and leave you feeling down. Keep it positive!

SUNDAY

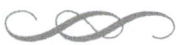

Morning Session

Find a quote, lyric, a picture, or something you have heard and stick it underneath. This is what you are going to start your day with! Make it funny or positive. Just as long as it makes you feel good. It is your dandelion in the concreate for the day!

Now write 5 goals that you want to achieve today. Remember you can make them small, medium or big, but make them achievable! Do not write things that you will not be able to achieve and whatever you cannot complete today does not roll over to tomorrow.

1. _____

   _____

2. _____

   _____

3. _____

   _____

4. _____

   _____

5. _____

   _____

Evening Session

Reflect on your day and now write 5 things or people that you are grateful for! Be Specific about your day. Remember you can be grateful for people, yourself or objects.

1. _____

_____

2. _____

_____

3. _____

_____

4. _____

_____

5. _____

_____

Has it been a hard day? This is where you write 5 things or people you want to forgive. Again, do not forget to be specific about the day! And remember you can include yourself, people or objects.

1. _____

_____

2. _____

_____

3. _____

_____

4. _____

_____

5. _____

_____

Reflection Space

This is your space! This is where you can make a few notes, you can do a spider diagram, you can doodle, or you can simply write down how you feel. If you are going to write down how you feel, remember to not rant and whine about your day, but to think of about, what you have learnt from the day and how you could improve for the next day. Ranting and moaning about the day will only create negative emotions and leave you feeling down. Keep it positive!

How to Sleep Better

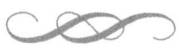

A good night's sleep can play an important role in good mental and physical health. It is an essential function that allows your body and mind to recharge and feel refreshed when we wake up in the morning. Without proper sleep, it could affect your concentration, memory, and cognitive thinking.

Studies have shown that an adult requires around seven to nine hours of sleep per night. However, there are many things in life that can affect a good night's sleep. The most common triggers are pressures that everyday life brings, such as work, family or relationship issues and although these may be short term, studies have shown that if sleep problems are not managed in the beginning, then they can persist long after the pressures have disappeared.

Over the years, people's sleep has deteriorated, and people are finding that they are sleeping less, and the quality of sleep is poorer. In the beginning, it may feel overwhelming, to look at your sleep pattern, but by simply making small simple changes, it could have a huge impact on your mental wellbeing.

In one study, it was shown that caffeine can stay elevated in your blood for 6 to 8 hours, therefore drinking drinks containing caffeine in the afternoon or close to bedtime could be disrupting your sleep. It is recommended to stop drinking caffeinated drinks after 3pm and maybe think about switching to water or herbal teas. If you really do want a coffee after 3pm, then consider a decaffeinated coffee instead. Also try not to drink a few hours going to before bed to prevent you from waking up in the middle of the night and wanting to use the toilet.

An hour before going to bed, it is good practice to try to disconnect from all devices. This is a good way to try and get your mind to relax and prepare for bed. This includes, phones, laptops, tablets and the television. Instead try reading a book or listening to some relaxing music.

Coming back from a hard day's work can leave our body feeling tense and we can still carry a lot of that tension when we are going to bed. One way of releasing that tension and helping our mind and body to prepare for bedtime is to have a nice bath, just before bed. It is also a good idea to infuse the bath with some lavender oil as there is much research that suggests that lavender is a natural product good for sleep problems.

Sometimes people cannot sleep because you might find yourself worrying about what has happened in the day or worried about tomorrow. If you have worries, get a notebook and write them down. When you write them down, it makes the worries real and stops them swirling around in your head. This may allow you to relax and sleep rather than have a disruptive night.

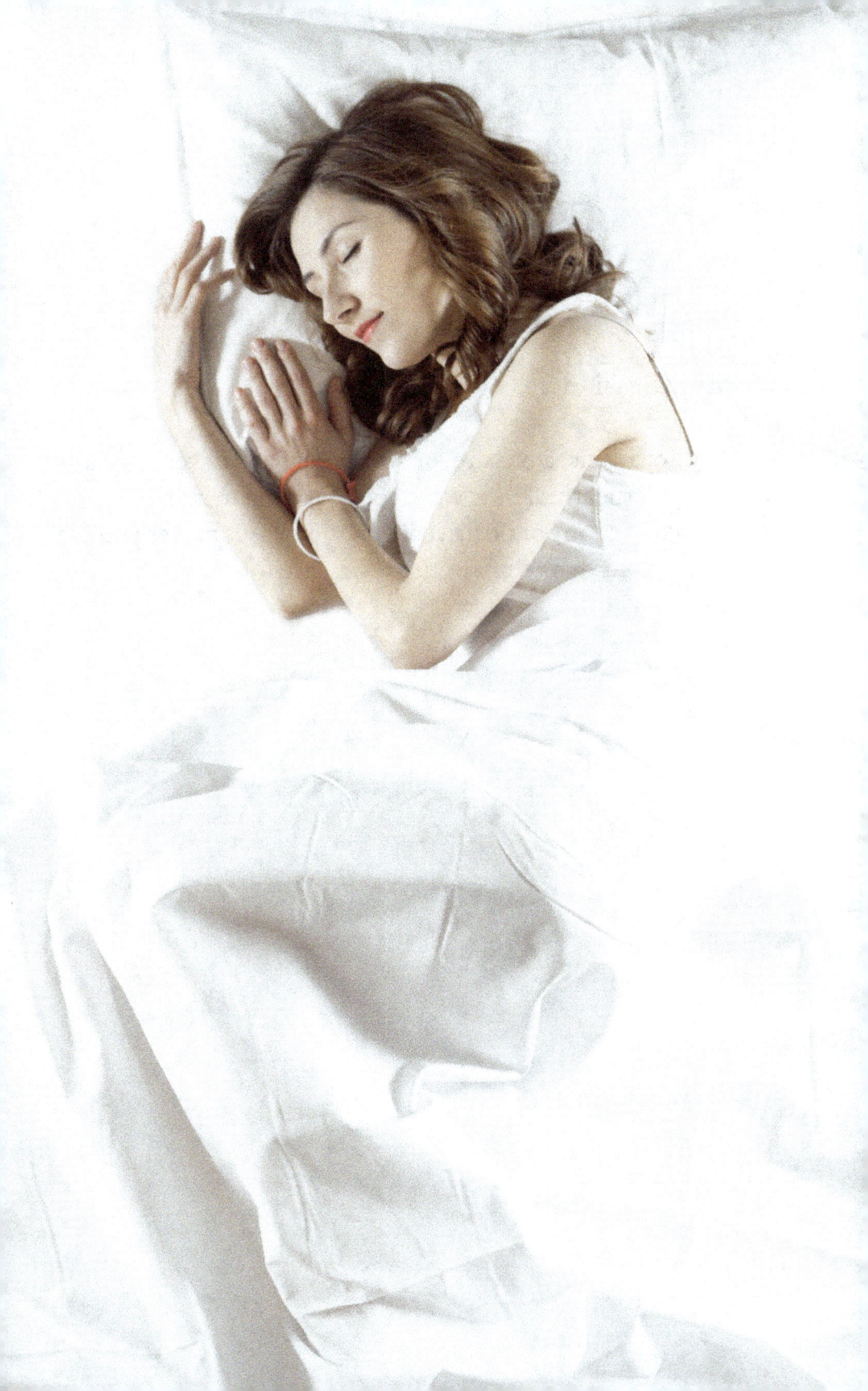

MONDAY

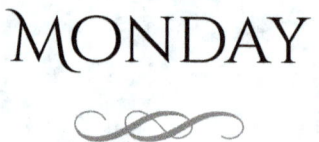

Morning Session

Find a quote, lyric, a picture, or something you have heard and stick it underneath. This is what you are going to start your day with! Make it funny or positive. Just as long as it makes you feel good. It is your dandelion in the concrete for the day!

Now write 5 goals that you want to achieve today. Remember you can make them small, medium or big, but make them achievable! Do not write things that you will not be able to achieve and whatever you cannot complete today does not roll over to tomorrow.

1. _____

   _____

2. _____

   _____

3. _____

   _____

4. _____

   _____

5. _____

   _____

   _____

Evening Session

Reflect on your day and now write 5 things or people that you are grateful for! Be Specific about your day. Remember you can be grateful for people, yourself or objects.

1. _____

_____

2. _____

_____

3. _____

_____

4. _____

_____

5. _____

_____

Has it been a hard day? This is where you write 5 things or people you want to forgive. Again, do not forget to be specific about the day! And remember you can include yourself, people or objects.

1. _____

   _____

2. _____

   _____

3. _____

   _____

4. _____

   _____

5. _____

   _____

Reflection Space

This is your space! This is where you can make a few notes, you can do a spider diagram, you can doodle, or you can simply write down how you feel. If you are going to write down how you feel, remember to not rant and whine about your day, but to think of about, what you have learnt from the day and how you could improve for the next day. Ranting and moaning about the day will only create negative emotions and leave you feeling down. Keep it positive!

TUESDAY

Morning Session

Find a quote, lyric, a picture, or something you have heard and stick it underneath. This is what you are going to start your day with! Make it funny or positive. Just as long as it makes you feel good. It is your dandelion in the concreate for the day!

Now write 5 goals that you want to achieve today. Remember you can make them small, medium or big, but make them achievable! Do not write things that you will not be able to achieve and whatever you cannot complete today does not roll over to tomorrow.

1. _____

   _____

2. _____

   _____

3. _____

   _____

4. _____

   _____

5. _____

   _____

Evening Session

Reflect on your day and now write 5 things or people that you are grateful for! Be Specific about your day. Remember you can be grateful for people, yourself or objects.

1. _____

   _____

2. _____

   _____

3. _____

   _____

4. _____

   _____

5. _____

   _____

Has it been a hard day? This is where you write 5 things or people you want to forgive. Again, do not forget to be specific about the day! And remember you can include yourself, people or objects.

1. _____

_____

2. _____

_____

3. _____

_____

4. _____

_____

5. _____

_____

Reflection Space

This is your space! This is where you can make a few notes, you can do a spider diagram, you can doodle, or you can simply write down how you feel. If you are going to write down how you feel, remember to not rant and whine about your day, but to think of about, what you have learnt from the day and how you could improve for the next day. Ranting and moaning about the day will only create negative emotions and leave you feeling down. Keep it positive!

WEDNESDAY

Morning Session

Find a quote, lyric, a picture, or something you have heard and stick it underneath. This is what you are going to start your day with! Make it funny or positive. Just as long as it makes you feel good. It is your dandelion in the concreate for the day!

Now write 5 goals that you want to achieve today. Remember you can make them small, medium or big, but make them achievable! Do not write things that you will not be able to achieve and whatever you cannot complete today does not roll over to tomorrow.

1. _____

   _____

2. _____

   _____

3. _____

   _____

4. _____

   _____

5. _____

   _____

Evening Session

Reflect on your day and now write 5 things or people that you are grateful for! Be Specific about your day. Remember you can be grateful for people, yourself or objects.

1. _____

_____

2. _____

_____

3. _____

_____

4. _____

_____

5. _____

_____

Has it been a hard day? This is where you write 5 things or people you want to forgive. Again, do not forget to be specific about the day! And remember you can include yourself, people or objects.

1. _____

   _____

2. _____

   _____

3. _____

   _____

4. _____

   _____

5. _____

   _____

Reflection Space

This is your space! This is where you can make a few notes, you can do a spider diagram, you can doodle, or you can simply write down how you feel. If you are going to write down how you feel, remember to not rant and whine about your day, but to think of about, what you have learnt from the day and how you could improve for the next day. Ranting and moaning about the day will only create negative emotions and leave you feeling down. Keep it positive!

THURSDAY

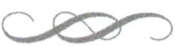

Morning Session

Find a quote, lyric, a picture, or something you have heard and stick it underneath. This is what you are going to start your day with! Make it funny or positive. Just as long as it makes you feel good. It is your dandelion in the concrete for the day!

Now write 5 goals that you want to achieve today. Remember you can make them small, medium or big, but make them achievable! Do not write things that you will not be able to achieve and whatever you cannot complete today does not roll over to tomorrow.

1. _____

   _____

2. _____

   _____

3. _____

   _____

4. _____

   _____

5. _____

   _____

Evening Session

Reflect on your day and now write 5 things or people that you are grateful for! Be Specific about your day. Remember you can be grateful for people, yourself or objects.

1. _____

_____

2. _____

_____

3. _____

_____

4. _____

_____

5. _____

_____

Has it been a hard day? This is where you write 5 things or people you want to forgive. Again, do not forget to be specific about the day! And remember you can include yourself, people or objects.

1. _____

_____

2. _____

_____

3. _____

_____

4. _____

_____

5. _____

_____

Reflection Space

This is your space! This is where you can make a few notes, you can do a spider diagram, you can doodle, or you can simply write down how you feel. If you are going to write down how you feel, remember to not rant and whine about your day, but to think of about, what you have learnt from the day and how you could improve for the next day. Ranting and moaning about the day will only create negative emotions and leave you feeling down. Keep it positive!

FRIDAY

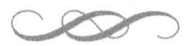

Morning Session

Find a quote, lyric, a picture, or something you have heard and stick it underneath. This is what you are going to start your day with! Make it funny or positive. Just as long as it makes you feel good. It is your dandelion in the concreate for the day!

Now write 5 goals that you want to achieve today. Remember you can make them small, medium or big, but make them achievable! Do not write things that you will not be able to achieve and whatever you cannot complete today does not roll over to tomorrow.

1. _____

   _____

2. _____

   _____

3. _____

   _____

4. _____

   _____

5. _____

   _____

Evening Session

Reflect on your day and now write 5 things or people that you are grateful for! Be Specific about your day. Remember you can be grateful for people, yourself or objects.

1. _____

   _____

2. _____

   _____

3. _____

   _____

4. _____

   _____

5. _____

   _____

Has it been a hard day? This is where you write 5 things or people you want to forgive. Again, do not forget to be specific about the day! And remember you can include yourself, people or objects.

1. _____

   _____

2. _____

   _____

3. _____

   _____

4. _____

   _____

5. _____

   _____

Reflection Space

This is your space! This is where you can make a few notes, you can do a spider diagram, you can doodle, or you can simply write down how you feel. If you are going to write down how you feel, remember to not rant and whine about your day, but to think of about, what you have learnt from the day and how you could improve for the next day. Ranting and moaning about the day will only create negative emotions and leave you feeling down. Keep it positive!

SATURDAY

Morning Session

Find a quote, lyric, a picture, or something you have heard and stick it underneath. This is what you are going to start your day with! Make it funny or positive. Just as long as it makes you feel good. It is your dandelion in the concreate for the day!

Now write 5 goals that you want to achieve today. Remember you can make them small, medium or big, but make them achievable! Do not write things that you will not be able to achieve and whatever you cannot complete today does not roll over to tomorrow.

1. _____

   _____

2. _____

   _____

3. _____

   _____

4. _____

   _____

5. _____

   _____

Evening Session

Reflect on your day and now write 5 things or people that you are grateful for! Be Specific about your day. Remember you can be grateful for people, yourself or objects.

1. _____

   _____

2. _____

   _____

3. _____

   _____

4. _____

   _____

5. _____

   _____

Has it been a hard day? This is where you write 5 things or people you want to forgive. Again, do not forget to be specific about the day! And remember you can include yourself, people or objects.

1. _____

_____

2. _____

_____

3. _____

_____

4. _____

_____

5. _____

_____

Reflection Space

This is your space! This is where you can make a few notes, you can do a spider diagram, you can doodle, or you can simply write down how you feel. If you are going to write down how you feel, remember to not rant and whine about your day, but to think of about, what you have learnt from the day and how you could improve for the next day. Ranting and moaning about the day will only create negative emotions and leave you feeling down. Keep it positive!

SUNDAY

Morning Session

Find a quote, lyric, a picture, or something you have heard and stick it underneath. This is what you are going to start your day with! Make it funny or positive. Just as long as it makes you feel good. It is your dandelion in the concreate for the day!

Now write 5 goals that you want to achieve today. Remember you can make them small, medium or big, but make them achievable! Do not write things that you will not be able to achieve and whatever you cannot complete today does not roll over to tomorrow.

1. _____

   _____

2. _____

   _____

3. _____

   _____

4. _____

   _____

5. _____

   _____

Evening Session

Reflect on your day and now write 5 things or people that you are grateful for! Be Specific about your day. Remember you can be grateful for people, yourself or objects.

1. _____

_____

2. _____

_____

3. _____

_____

4. _____

_____

5. _____

_____

Has it been a hard day? This is where you write 5 things or people you want to forgive. Again, do not forget to be specific about the day! And remember you can include yourself, people or objects.

1. _____

   _____

2. _____

   _____

3. _____

   _____

4. _____

   _____

5. _____

   _____

Reflection Space

This is your space! This is where you can make a few notes, you can do a spider diagram, you can doodle, or you can simply write down how you feel. If you are going to write down how you feel, remember to not rant and whine about your day, but to think of about, what you have learnt from the day and how you could improve for the next day. Ranting and moaning about the day will only create negative emotions and leave you feeling down. Keep it positive!

STRESS MANAGEMENT

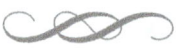

Life can be stressful at times and although a small amount of stress is good for you because it can motivate you, too much stress can cause havoc with our emotional wellbeing.

When your body is under quite a lot of stress. Our body feels under attack and automatically goes into a physical response of fight and flight mode. Back when we were cavemen and cavewomen, this fight and flight mode came in handy, as it alerted us to danger. The release of hormones such as adrenaline, cortisol and norepinephrine prepared us to either fight the danger or to run away from it. The world around us has evolved but our bodies have not, which means that when we go into a state of stress, our bodies still release the hormones, but in the modern world we have nothing to fight or run away from so therefore we have no way of bringing the hormones down from our system. This means that the hormones stay elevated in our system which becomes detrimental to our health. Therefore, when blood flow is going only to the most important muscles needed to fight and flight, the brain function is minimised. This can then lead to an inability to think straight and can leave you feeling fatigued. Also, the high level of cortisol can increase your blood pressure and can decrease libido.

There are many things that you can put in place to help you manage your stress better in everyday life. One of the most important things you could do is manage your time effectively. Time management is crucial in today's busy society. When you do not manage your time effectively, it is easy to cut back on your own health. Make sure you do not over commit yourself and do not forget to schedule in leisure activities as this is a great way to relieve stress and have fun.

When thinking about stress, it is good to try and identify what the sources of your stresses are. Once you have identified your source of stress, you may want to try to eliminate them or even minimise them. However, there may be certain situations that you might not be able to change, but you will be able to choose how you react to those situations.

It is important to remember that you cannot do things perfectly no matter how hard you try. Remember that you will not be able to control everything in your life and life is for living and making memories, so go and make memories and live life and try not to stress about the things you cannot change.

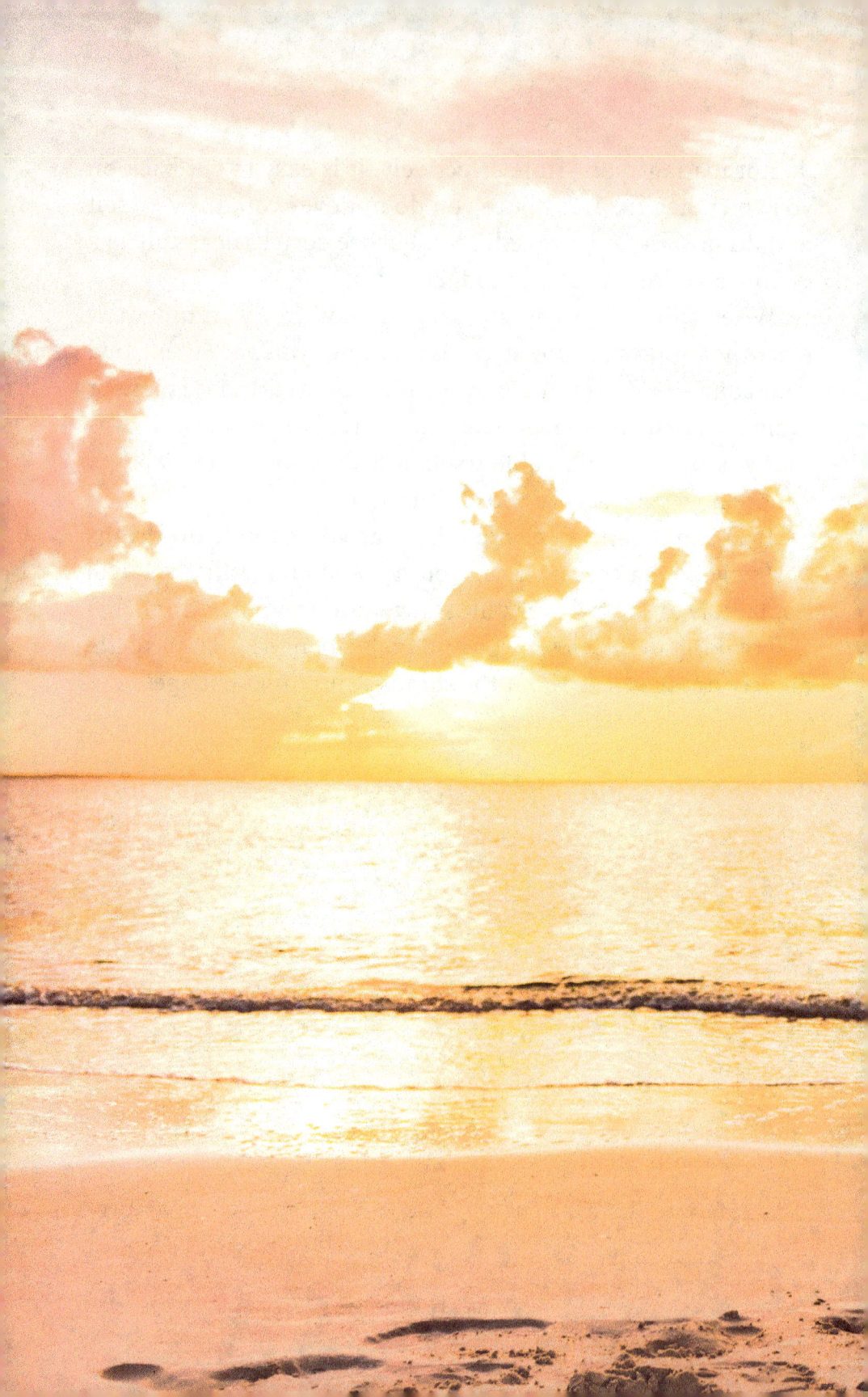

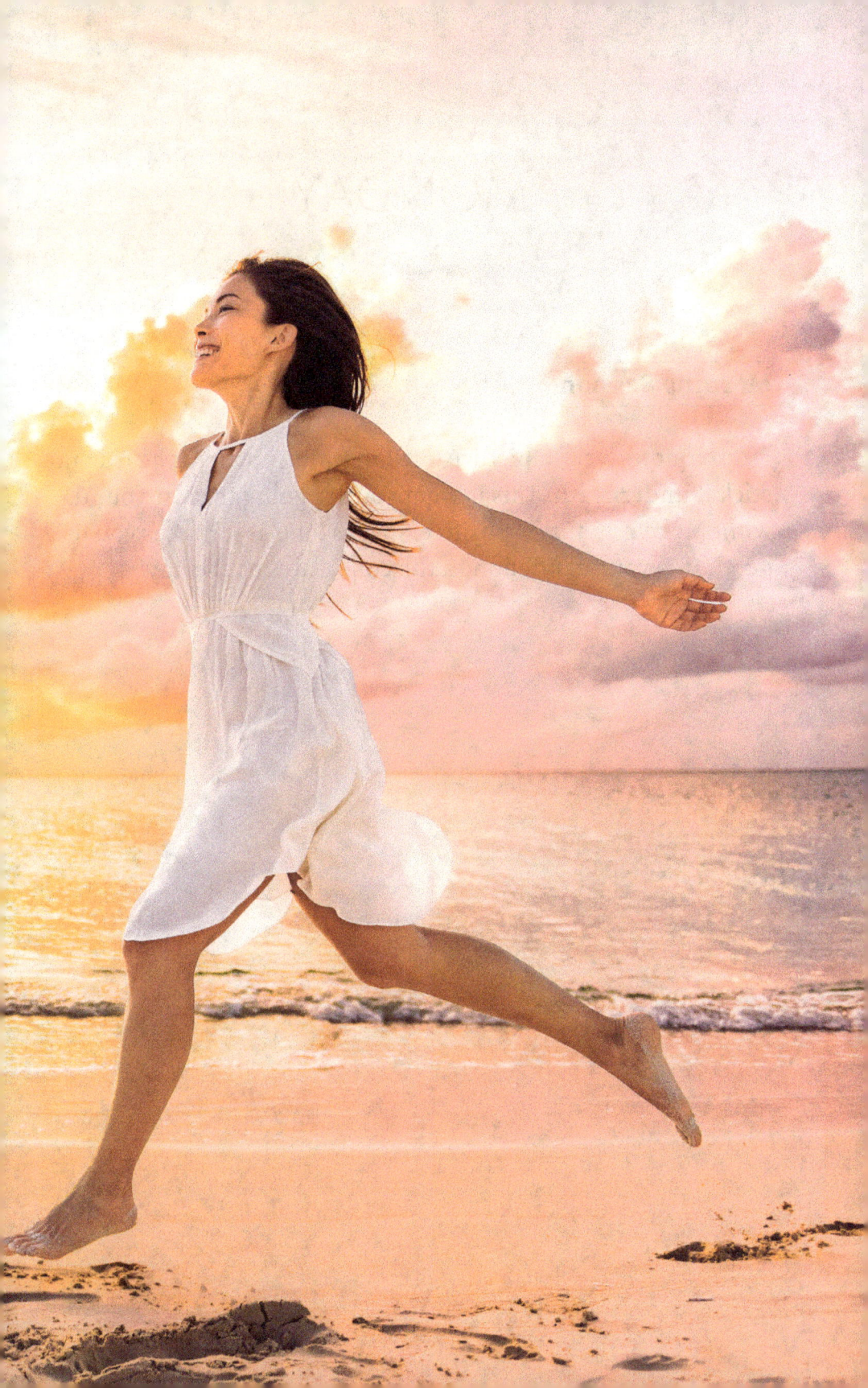

MONDAY

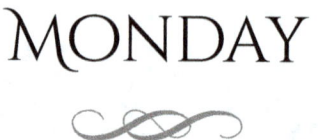

Morning Session

Find a quote, lyric, a picture, or something you have heard and stick it underneath. This is what you are going to start your day with! Make it funny or positive. Just as long as it makes you feel good. It is your dandelion in the concreate for the day!

Now write 5 goals that you want to achieve today. Remember you can make them small, medium or big, but make them achievable! Do not write things that you will not be able to achieve and whatever you cannot complete today does not roll over to tomorrow.

1. _____

   _____

2. _____

   _____

3. _____

   _____

4. _____

   _____

5. _____

   _____

Evening Session

Reflect on your day and now write 5 things or people that you are grateful for! Be Specific about your day. Remember you can be grateful for people, yourself or objects.

1. _____

   _____

2. _____

   _____

3. _____

   _____

4. _____

   _____

5. _____

   _____

Has it been a hard day? This is where you write 5 things or people you want to forgive. Again, do not forget to be specific about the day! And remember you can include yourself, people or objects.

1. _____

   _____

2. _____

   _____

3. _____

   _____

4. _____

   _____

5. _____

   _____

Reflection Space

This is your space! This is where you can make a few notes, you can do a spider diagram, you can doodle, or you can simply write down how you feel. If you are going to write down how you feel, remember to not rant and whine about your day, but to think of about, what you have learnt from the day and how you could improve for the next day. Ranting and moaning about the day will only create negative emotions and leave you feeling down. Keep it positive!

TUESDAY

Morning Session

Find a quote, lyric, a picture, or something you have heard and stick it underneath. This is what you are going to start your day with! Make it funny or positive. Just as long as it makes you feel good. It is your dandelion in the concreate for the day!

Now write 5 goals that you want to achieve today. Remember you can make them small, medium or big, but make them achievable! Do not write things that you will not be able to achieve and whatever you cannot complete today does not roll over to tomorrow.

1. _____

   _____

2. _____

   _____

3. _____

   _____

4. _____

   _____

5. _____

   _____

Evening Session

Reflect on your day and now write 5 things or people that you are grateful for! Be Specific about your day. Remember you can be grateful for people, yourself or objects.

1. _____

_____

2. _____

_____

3. _____

_____

4. _____

_____

5. _____

_____

Has it been a hard day? This is where you write 5 things or people you want to forgive. Again, do not forget to be specific about the day! And remember you can include yourself, people or objects.

1. _____

   _____

2. _____

   _____

3. _____

   _____

4. _____

   _____

5. _____

   _____

Reflection Space

This is your space! This is where you can make a few notes, you can do a spider diagram, you can doodle, or you can simply write down how you feel. If you are going to write down how you feel, remember to not rant and whine about your day, but to think of about, what you have learnt from the day and how you could improve for the next day. Ranting and moaning about the day will only create negative emotions and leave you feeling down. Keep it positive!

WEDNESDAY

Morning Session

Find a quote, lyric, a picture, or something you have heard and stick it underneath. This is what you are going to start your day with! Make it funny or positive. Just as long as it makes you feel good. It is your dandelion in the concreate for the day!

Now write 5 goals that you want to achieve today. Remember you can make them small, medium or big, but make them achievable! Do not write things that you will not be able to achieve and whatever you cannot complete today does not roll over to tomorrow.

1. _____

   _____

2. _____

   _____

3. _____

   _____

4. _____

   _____

5. _____

   _____

Evening Session

Reflect on your day and now write 5 things or people that you are grateful for! Be Specific about your day. Remember you can be grateful for people, yourself or objects.

1. _____

_____

2. _____

_____

3. _____

_____

4. _____

_____

5. _____

_____

Has it been a hard day? This is where you write 5 things or people you want to forgive. Again, do not forget to be specific about the day! And remember you can include yourself, people or objects.

1. _____

_____

2. _____

_____

3. _____

_____

4. _____

_____

5. _____

_____

Reflection Space

This is your space! This is where you can make a few notes, you can do a spider diagram, you can doodle, or you can simply write down how you feel. If you are going to write down how you feel, remember to not rant and whine about your day, but to think of about, what you have learnt from the day and how you could improve for the next day. Ranting and moaning about the day will only create negative emotions and leave you feeling down. Keep it positive!

THURSDAY

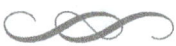

Morning Session

Find a quote, lyric, a picture, or something you have heard and stick it underneath. This is what you are going to start your day with! Make it funny or positive. Just as long as it makes you feel good. It is your dandelion in the concreate for the day!

Now write 5 goals that you want to achieve today. Remember you can make them small, medium or big, but make them achievable! Do not write things that you will not be able to achieve and whatever you cannot complete today does not roll over to tomorrow.

1. _____

   _____

2. _____

   _____

3. _____

   _____

4. _____

   _____

5. _____

   _____

Evening Session

Reflect on your day and now write 5 things or people that you are grateful for! Be Specific about your day. Remember you can be grateful for people, yourself or objects.

1. _____

   _____

2. _____

   _____

3. _____

   _____

4. _____

   _____

5. _____

   _____

Has it been a hard day? This is where you write 5 things or people you want to forgive. Again, do not forget to be specific about the day! And remember you can include yourself, people or objects.

1. _____
   _____

2. _____
   _____

3. _____
   _____

4. _____
   _____

5. _____
   _____

Reflection Space

This is your space! This is where you can make a few notes, you can do a spider diagram, you can doodle, or you can simply write down how you feel. If you are going to write down how you feel, remember to not rant and whine about your day, but to think of about, what you have learnt from the day and how you could improve for the next day. Ranting and moaning about the day will only create negative emotions and leave you feeling down. Keep it positive!

FRIDAY

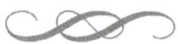

Morning Session

Find a quote, lyric, a picture, or something you have heard and stick it underneath. This is what you are going to start your day with! Make it funny or positive. Just as long as it makes you feel good. It is your dandelion in the concreate for the day!

Now write 5 goals that you want to achieve today. Remember you can make them small, medium or big, but make them achievable! Do not write things that you will not be able to achieve and whatever you cannot complete today does not roll over to tomorrow.

1. _____

   _____

2. _____

   _____

3. _____

   _____

4. _____

   _____

5. _____

   _____

Evening Session

Reflect on your day and now write 5 things or people that you are grateful for! Be Specific about your day. Remember you can be grateful for people, yourself or objects.

1. _____

   _____

2. _____

   _____

3. _____

   _____

4. _____

   _____

5. _____

   _____

Has it been a hard day? This is where you write 5 things or people you want to forgive. Again, do not forget to be specific about the day! And remember you can include yourself, people or objects.

1. _____

   _____

2. _____

   _____

3. _____

   _____

4. _____

   _____

5. _____

   _____

Reflection Space

This is your space! This is where you can make a few notes, you can do a spider diagram, you can doodle, or you can simply write down how you feel. If you are going to write down how you feel, remember to not rant and whine about your day, but to think of about, what you have learnt from the day and how you could improve for the next day. Ranting and moaning about the day will only create negative emotions and leave you feeling down. Keep it positive!

SATURDAY

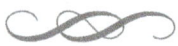

Morning Session

Find a quote, lyric, a picture, or something you have heard and stick it underneath. This is what you are going to start your day with! Make it funny or positive. Just as long as it makes you feel good. It is your dandelion in the concreate for the day!

Now write 5 goals that you want to achieve today. Remember you can make them small, medium or big, but make them achievable! Do not write things that you will not be able to achieve and whatever you cannot complete today does not roll over to tomorrow.

1. _____

   _____

2. _____

   _____

3. _____

   _____

4. _____

   _____

5. _____

   _____

Evening Session

Reflect on your day and now write 5 things or people that you are grateful for! Be Specific about your day. Remember you can be grateful for people, yourself or objects.

1. _____

_____

2. _____

_____

3. _____

_____

4. _____

_____

5. _____

_____

Has it been a hard day? This is where you write 5 things or people you want to forgive. Again, do not forget to be specific about the day! And remember you can include yourself, people or objects.

1. _____

   _____

2. _____

   _____

3. _____

   _____

4. _____

   _____

5. _____

   _____

Reflection Space

This is your space! This is where you can make a few notes, you can do a spider diagram, you can doodle, or you can simply write down how you feel. If you are going to write down how you feel, remember to not rant and whine about your day, but to think of about, what you have learnt from the day and how you could improve for the next day. Ranting and moaning about the day will only create negative emotions and leave you feeling down. Keep it positive!

SUNDAY

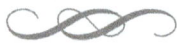

Morning Session

Find a quote, lyric, a picture, or something you have heard and stick it underneath. This is what you are going to start your day with! Make it funny or positive. Just as long as it makes you feel good. It is your dandelion in the concreate for the day!

Now write 5 goals that you want to achieve today. Remember you can make them small, medium or big, but make them achievable! Do not write things that you will not be able to achieve and whatever you cannot complete today does not roll over to tomorrow.

1. _____

   _____

2. _____

   _____

3. _____

   _____

4. _____

   _____

5. _____

   _____

Evening Session

Reflect on your day and now write 5 things or people that you are grateful for! Be Specific about your day. Remember you can be grateful for people, yourself or objects.

1. _____

_____

2. _____

_____

3. _____

_____

4. _____

_____

5. _____

_____

Has it been a hard day? This is where you write 5 things or people you want to forgive. Again, do not forget to be specific about the day! And remember you can include yourself, people or objects.

1. _____

   _____

2. _____

   _____

3. _____

   _____

4. _____

   _____

5. _____

   _____

Reflection Space

This is your space! This is where you can make a few notes, you can do a spider diagram, you can doodle, or you can simply write down how you feel. If you are going to write down how you feel, remember to not rant and whine about your day, but to think of about, what you have learnt from the day and how you could improve for the next day. Ranting and moaning about the day will only create negative emotions and leave you feeling down. Keep it positive!

HOW TO OVERCOME FEAR

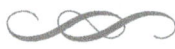

Fears and anxieties are a normal part of life and most people will have some sort of fear or anxiety, such as spiders, flying or going to the dentist. When these fears and anxieties start to interfere with everyday life, it can cause huge problems, affecting your eating, sleeping and concentration.

When you are feeling anxious, you may experience uncomfortable thoughts as well as physical symptoms. The physical symptoms alone can be very scary, such as a racing heart and the feeling of suffocation, but by learning how to calm yourself down can help you to not make these symptoms any worse.

One way of managing fear is by confronting your fear. Each time you confront your fear, you would reduce your reaction to your fear therefore either learning to manage the fear or completely eradicating the fear.

Another way you can manage your fears is by using visualizing techniques. You can imagine a place of safety and calm. This could be a picture of an exotic place that you have been or want to visit or it could be a place where you feel safe and happy. Once you embrace those positive feelings, you might find yourself letting go of your fears and anxieties.

When you have fears or anxieties, you may even have negative thoughts, which can give you a distorted view of yourself and the world. It can sometimes help to identify those irrational thoughts and then challenge those thoughts. One way of doing this is by writing down your worries and then looking at the worst-case scenario. By writing it down and thinking of the worst-case scenario, you might find that your fears were not that bad, or you might find that they were manageable.

Life is full of stresses, yet many of us feel that our lives must be perfect. Bad days and setbacks are evitable and its important to remember that life has its ups and downs. However, when you have these ups and down, remember to be kind and gentle to yourself. True compassion is about being able to understand ones suffering and from that we are able to make the changes that we need to make, whether those changes are in the external world or whether they are changes in your responses to the external world.

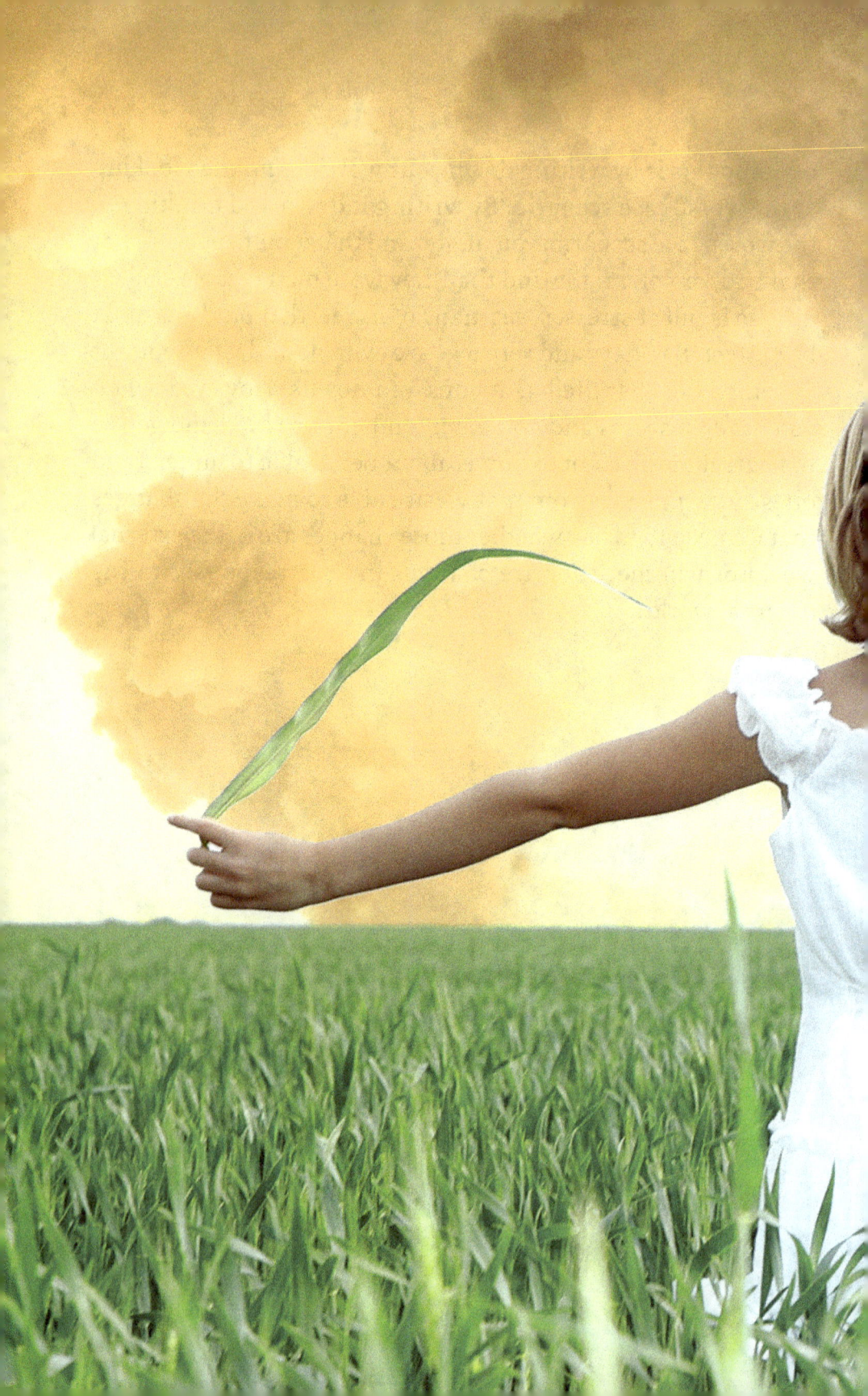

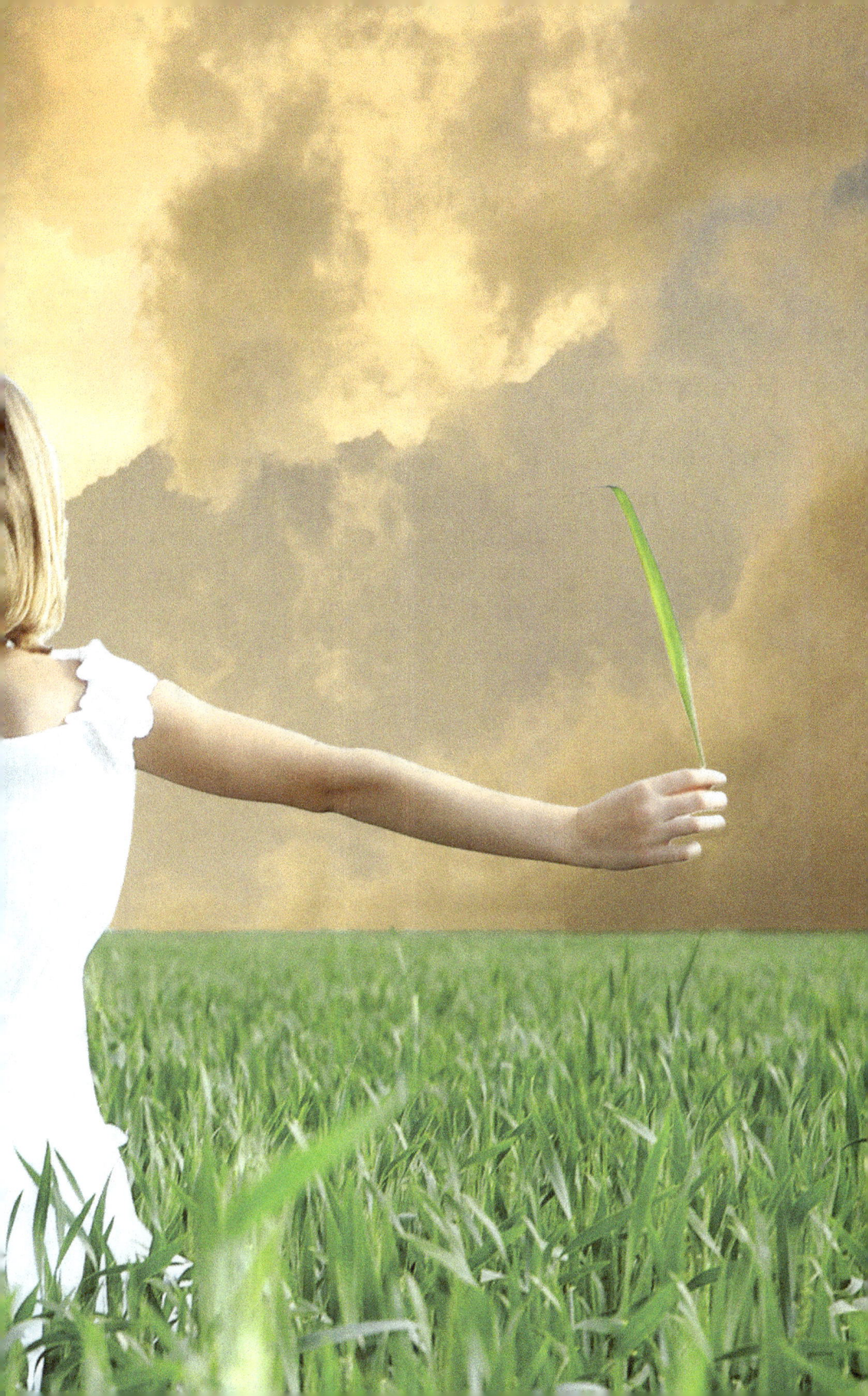

MONDAY

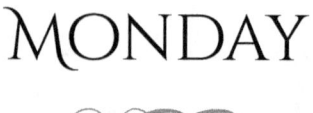

Morning Session

Find a quote, lyric, a picture, or something you have heard and stick it underneath. This is what you are going to start your day with! Make it funny or positive. Just as long as it makes you feel good. It is your dandelion in the concreate for the day!

Now write 5 goals that you want to achieve today. Remember you can make them small, medium or big, but make them achievable! Do not write things that you will not be able to achieve and whatever you cannot complete today does not roll over to tomorrow.

1. _____

   _____

2. _____

   _____

3. _____

   _____

4. _____

   _____

5. _____

   _____

Evening Session

Reflect on your day and now write 5 things or people that you are grateful for! Be Specific about your day. Remember you can be grateful for people, yourself or objects.

1. _____

   _____

2. _____

   _____

3. _____

   _____

4. _____

   _____

5. _____

   _____

Has it been a hard day? This is where you write 5 things or people you want to forgive. Again, do not forget to be specific about the day! And remember you can include yourself, people or objects.

1. _____

   _____

2. _____

   _____

3. _____

   _____

4. _____

   _____

5. _____

   _____

Reflection Space

This is your space! This is where you can make a few notes, you can do a spider diagram, you can doodle, or you can simply write down how you feel. If you are going to write down how you feel, remember to not rant and whine about your day, but to think of about, what you have learnt from the day and how you could improve for the next day. Ranting and moaning about the day will only create negative emotions and leave you feeling down. Keep it positive!

TUESDAY

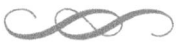

Morning Session

Find a quote, lyric, a picture, or something you have heard and stick it underneath. This is what you are going to start your day with! Make it funny or positive. Just as long as it makes you feel good. It is your dandelion in the concreate for the day!

Now write 5 goals that you want to achieve today. Remember you can make them small, medium or big, but make them achievable! Do not write things that you will not be able to achieve and whatever you cannot complete today does not roll over to tomorrow.

1. _____

   _____

2. _____

   _____

3. _____

   _____

4. _____

   _____

5. _____

   _____

Evening Session

Reflect on your day and now write 5 things or people that you are grateful for! Be Specific about your day. Remember you can be grateful for people, yourself or objects.

1. _____

_____

2. _____

_____

3. _____

_____

4. _____

_____

5. _____

_____

Has it been a hard day? This is where you write 5 things or people you want to forgive. Again, do not forget to be specific about the day! And remember you can include yourself, people or objects.

1. _____

   _____

2. _____

   _____

3. _____

   _____

4. _____

   _____

5. _____

   _____

Reflection Space

This is your space! This is where you can make a few notes, you can do a spider diagram, you can doodle, or you can simply write down how you feel. If you are going to write down how you feel, remember to not rant and whine about your day, but to think of about, what you have learnt from the day and how you could improve for the next day. Ranting and moaning about the day will only create negative emotions and leave you feeling down. Keep it positive!

WEDNESDAY

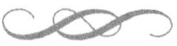

Morning Session

Find a quote, lyric, a picture, or something you have heard and stick it underneath. This is what you are going to start your day with! Make it funny or positive. Just as long as it makes you feel good. It is your dandelion in the concreate for the day!

Now write 5 goals that you want to achieve today. Remember you can make them small, medium or big, but make them achievable! Do not write things that you will not be able to achieve and whatever you cannot complete today does not roll over to tomorrow.

1. _____

   _____

2. _____

   _____

3. _____

   _____

4. _____

   _____

5. _____

   _____

Evening Session

Reflect on your day and now write 5 things or people that you are grateful for! Be Specific about your day. Remember you can be grateful for people, yourself or objects.

1. _____

_____

2. _____

_____

3. _____

_____

4. _____

_____

5. _____

_____

Has it been a hard day? This is where you write 5 things or people you want to forgive. Again, do not forget to be specific about the day! And remember you can include yourself, people or objects.

1. _____

   _____

2. _____

   _____

3. _____

   _____

4. _____

   _____

5. _____

   _____

Reflection Space

This is your space! This is where you can make a few notes, you can do a spider diagram, you can doodle, or you can simply write down how you feel. If you are going to write down how you feel, remember to not rant and whine about your day, but to think of about, what you have learnt from the day and how you could improve for the next day. Ranting and moaning about the day will only create negative emotions and leave you feeling down. Keep it positive!

THURSDAY

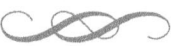

Morning Session

Find a quote, lyric, a picture, or something you have heard and stick it underneath. This is what you are going to start your day with! Make it funny or positive. Just as long as it makes you feel good. It is your dandelion in the concreate for the day!

Now write 5 goals that you want to achieve today. Remember you can make them small, medium or big, but make them achievable! Do not write things that you will not be able to achieve and whatever you cannot complete today does not roll over to tomorrow.

1. _____

   _____

2. _____

   _____

3. _____

   _____

4. _____

   _____

5. _____

   _____

Evening Session

Reflect on your day and now write 5 things or people that you are grateful for! Be Specific about your day. Remember you can be grateful for people, yourself or objects.

1. _____

   _____

2. _____

   _____

3. _____

   _____

4. _____

   _____

5. _____

   _____

Has it been a hard day? This is where you write 5 things or people you want to forgive. Again, do not forget to be specific about the day! And remember you can include yourself, people or objects.

1. _____

   _____

2. _____

   _____

3. _____

   _____

4. _____

   _____

5. _____

   _____

Reflection Space

This is your space! This is where you can make a few notes, you can do a spider diagram, you can doodle, or you can simply write down how you feel. If you are going to write down how you feel, remember to not rant and whine about your day, but to think of about, what you have learnt from the day and how you could improve for the next day. Ranting and moaning about the day will only create negative emotions and leave you feeling down. Keep it positive!

FRIDAY

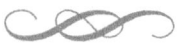

Morning Session

Find a quote, lyric, a picture, or something you have heard and stick it underneath. This is what you are going to start your day with! Make it funny or positive. Just as long as it makes you feel good. It is your dandelion in the concreate for the day!

Now write 5 goals that you want to achieve today. Remember you can make them small, medium or big, but make them achievable! Do not write things that you will not be able to achieve and whatever you cannot complete today does not roll over to tomorrow.

1. _____

   _____

2. _____

   _____

3. _____

   _____

4. _____

   _____

5. _____

   _____

Evening Session

Reflect on your day and now write 5 things or people that you are grateful for! Be Specific about your day. Remember you can be grateful for people, yourself or objects.

1. _____

   _____

2. _____

   _____

3. _____

   _____

4. _____

   _____

5. _____

   _____

Has it been a hard day? This is where you write 5 things or people you want to forgive. Again, do not forget to be specific about the day! And remember you can include yourself, people or objects.

1. _____

   _____

2. _____

   _____

3. _____

   _____

4. _____

   _____

5. _____

   _____

Reflection Space

This is your space! This is where you can make a few notes, you can do a spider diagram, you can doodle, or you can simply write down how you feel. If you are going to write down how you feel, remember to not rant and whine about your day, but to think of about, what you have learnt from the day and how you could improve for the next day. Ranting and moaning about the day will only create negative emotions and leave you feeling down. Keep it positive!

SATURDAY

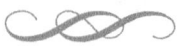

Morning Session

Find a quote, lyric, a picture, or something you have heard and stick it underneath. This is what you are going to start your day with! Make it funny or positive. Just as long as it makes you feel good. It is your dandelion in the concreate for the day!

Now write 5 goals that you want to achieve today. Remember you can make them small, medium or big, but make them achievable! Do not write things that you will not be able to achieve and whatever you cannot complete today does not roll over to tomorrow.

1. _____

   _____

2. _____

   _____

3. _____

   _____

4. _____

   _____

5. _____

   _____

Evening Session

Reflect on your day and now write 5 things or people that you are grateful for! Be Specific about your day. Remember you can be grateful for people, yourself or objects.

1. _____

   _____

2. _____

   _____

3. _____

   _____

4. _____

   _____

5. _____

   _____

Has it been a hard day? This is where you write 5 things or people you want to forgive. Again, do not forget to be specific about the day! And remember you can include yourself, people or objects.

1. _____

   _____

2. _____

   _____

3. _____

   _____

4. _____

   _____

5. _____

   _____

Reflection Space

This is your space! This is where you can make a few notes, you can do a spider diagram, you can doodle, or you can simply write down how you feel. If you are going to write down how you feel, remember to not rant and whine about your day, but to think of about, what you have learnt from the day and how you could improve for the next day. Ranting and moaning about the day will only create negative emotions and leave you feeling down. Keep it positive!

SUNDAY

Morning Session

Find a quote, lyric, a picture, or something you have heard and stick it underneath. This is what you are going to start your day with! Make it funny or positive. Just as long as it makes you feel good. It is your dandelion in the concreate for the day!

Now write 5 goals that you want to achieve today. Remember you can make them small, medium or big, but make them achievable! Do not write things that you will not be able to achieve and whatever you cannot complete today does not roll over to tomorrow.

1. _____

   _____

2. _____

   _____

3. _____

   _____

4. _____

   _____

5. _____

   _____

Evening Session

Reflect on your day and now write 5 things or people that you are grateful for! Be Specific about your day. Remember you can be grateful for people, yourself or objects.

1. _____

   _____

2. _____

   _____

3. _____

   _____

4. _____

   _____

5. _____

   _____

Has it been a hard day? This is where you write 5 things or people you want to forgive. Again, do not forget to be specific about the day! And remember you can include yourself, people or objects.

1. _____

_____

2. _____

_____

3. _____

_____

4. _____

_____

5. _____

_____

Reflection Space

This is your space! This is where you can make a few notes, you can do a spider diagram, you can doodle, or you can simply write down how you feel. If you are going to write down how you feel, remember to not rant and whine about your day, but to think of about, what you have learnt from the day and how you could improve for the next day. Ranting and moaning about the day will only create negative emotions and leave you feeling down. Keep it positive!

SELF DISCIPLINE

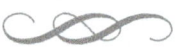

You can do many things that pertain to your happiness and inner peace, but one is thing that is crucial to keeping this up long term, is self-discipline. Self-discipline is the ability that you have to push forward, stay motivated and act, regardless of how you are feeling, physically or emotionally. Becoming Self-disciplined, despite what you may think and believe is a learned behaviour that we can develop. Therefore, it requires practice and repetition in everyday life, for you to improve.

When trying to maintain self-discipline, it is important that you do not set unrealistic goals for yourself. Make sure your goals are small and achievable. When you set big goals that are unachievable, you can become overwhelmed by them and then they can become intimidating. Give yourself time and be patient and kind with yourself and most of all be realistic with yourself setting realistic timeframes.

Do not forget that there are victories in everything, even with your failures and make sure you celebrate them. When you fail at something, you learn from it and you know what to do differently next time. Every time you fail, it is important to note that you now have new knowledge that can help you to improve what you are doing. It also means that you have given something a try which is better than not giving it try at all. Whether you fail or you succeed, you are a winner. Hold on to that!

Sometimes being disciplined can seem long and arduous and rewards can seem far away. During these times, you need to remind yourself of the reason why you are making these changes. You can do this two ways, One way is by writing down a list of all the things that you are going to gain from sticking to your goals and another way is to create a vision board where you would create a board full of pictures of what you want to achieve with the goals. Then you would place them somewhere that you could view them on a regular basis so that you could keep focused.

Remember when trying to keep self-disciplined, you do not have to do it alone. You can ask for help from family and friends and people around you. Gathering people around you can be the best way to help you keep self-disciplined and can make it fun rather than making it a chore. After all self-love and self-care is all about having fun and enjoying life, not making it another burden in life. It is about appreciating you and others you and making the most of life as we know it.

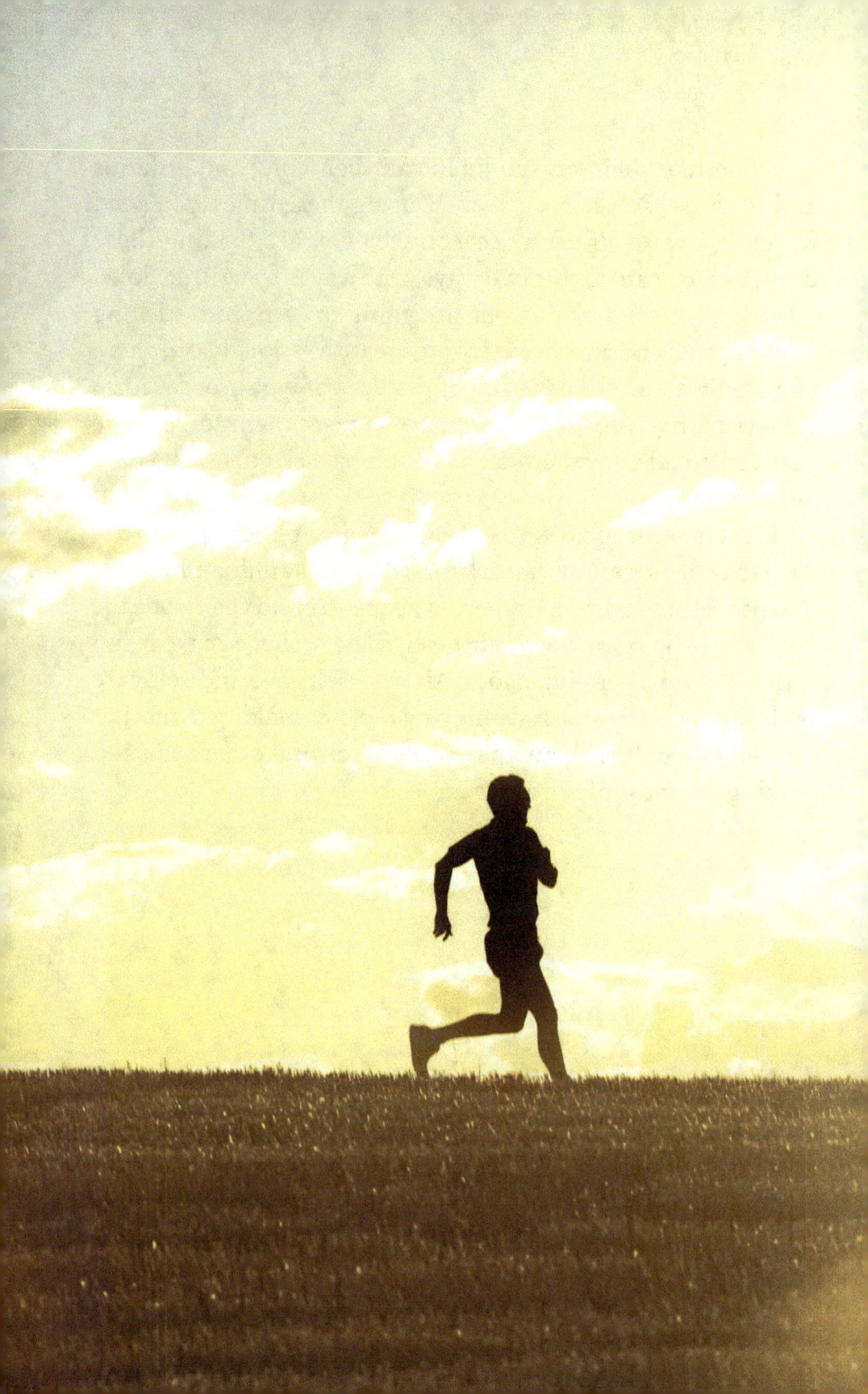

MONDAY

Morning Session

Find a quote, lyric, a picture, or something you have heard and stick it underneath. This is what you are going to start your day with! Make it funny or positive. Just as long as it makes you feel good. It is your dandelion in the concreate for the day!

Now write 5 goals that you want to achieve today. Remember you can make them small, medium or big, but make them achievable! Do not write things that you will not be able to achieve and whatever you cannot complete today does not roll over to tomorrow.

1. _____

   _____

2. _____

   _____

3. _____

   _____

4. _____

   _____

5. _____

   _____

Evening Session

Reflect on your day and now write 5 things or people that you are grateful for! Be Specific about your day. Remember you can be grateful for people, yourself or objects.

1. _____

_____

2. _____

_____

3. _____

_____

4. _____

_____

5. _____

_____

Has it been a hard day? This is where you write 5 things or people you want to forgive. Again, do not forget to be specific about the day! And remember you can include yourself, people or objects.

1. _____

   _____

2. _____

   _____

3. _____

   _____

4. _____

   _____

5. _____

   _____

Reflection Space

This is your space! This is where you can make a few notes, you can do a spider diagram, you can doodle, or you can simply write down how you feel. If you are going to write down how you feel, remember to not rant and whine about your day, but to think of about, what you have learnt from the day and how you could improve for the next day. Ranting and moaning about the day will only create negative emotions and leave you feeling down. Keep it positive!

TUESDAY

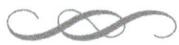

Morning Session

Find a quote, lyric, a picture, or something you have heard and stick it underneath. This is what you are going to start your day with! Make it funny or positive. Just as long as it makes you feel good. It is your dandelion in the concreate for the day!

Now write 5 goals that you want to achieve today. Remember you can make them small, medium or big, but make them achievable! Do not write things that you will not be able to achieve and whatever you cannot complete today does not roll over to tomorrow.

1. _____

   _____

2. _____

   _____

3. _____

   _____

4. _____

   _____

5. _____

   _____

Evening Session

Reflect on your day and now write 5 things or people that you are grateful for! Be Specific about your day. Remember you can be grateful for people, yourself or objects.

1. _____

_____

2. _____

_____

3. _____

_____

4. _____

_____

5. _____

_____

Has it been a hard day? This is where you write 5 things or people you want to forgive. Again, do not forget to be specific about the day! And remember you can include yourself, people or objects.

1. _____

   _____

2. _____

   _____

3. _____

   _____

4. _____

   _____

5. _____

   _____

Reflection Space

This is your space! This is where you can make a few notes, you can do a spider diagram, you can doodle, or you can simply write down how you feel. If you are going to write down how you feel, remember to not rant and whine about your day, but to think of about, what you have learnt from the day and how you could improve for the next day. Ranting and moaning about the day will only create negative emotions and leave you feeling down. Keep it positive!

WEDNESDAY

Morning Session

Find a quote, lyric, a picture, or something you have heard and stick it underneath. This is what you are going to start your day with! Make it funny or positive. Just as long as it makes you feel good. It is your dandelion in the concreate for the day!

Now write 5 goals that you want to achieve today. Remember you can make them small, medium or big, but make them achievable! Do not write things that you will not be able to achieve and whatever you cannot complete today does not roll over to tomorrow.

1. _____

   _____

2. _____

   _____

3. _____

   _____

4. _____

   _____

5. _____

   _____

Evening Session

Reflect on your day and now write 5 things or people that you are grateful for! Be Specific about your day. Remember you can be grateful for people, yourself or objects.

1. _____

   _____

2. _____

   _____

3. _____

   _____

4. _____

   _____

5. _____

   _____

Has it been a hard day? This is where you write 5 things or people you want to forgive. Again, do not forget to be specific about the day! And remember you can include yourself, people or objects.

1. _____

   _____

2. _____

   _____

3. _____

   _____

4. _____

   _____

5. _____

   _____

Reflection Space

This is your space! This is where you can make a few notes, you can do a spider diagram, you can doodle, or you can simply write down how you feel. If you are going to write down how you feel, remember to not rant and whine about your day, but to think of about, what you have learnt from the day and how you could improve for the next day. Ranting and moaning about the day will only create negative emotions and leave you feeling down. Keep it positive!

THURSDAY

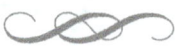

Morning Session

Find a quote, lyric, a picture, or something you have heard and stick it underneath. This is what you are going to start your day with! Make it funny or positive. Just as long as it makes you feel good. It is your dandelion in the concreate for the day!

Now write 5 goals that you want to achieve today. Remember you can make them small, medium or big, but make them achievable! Do not write things that you will not be able to achieve and whatever you cannot complete today does not roll over to tomorrow.

1. _____

   _____

2. _____

   _____

3. _____

   _____

4. _____

   _____

5. _____

   _____

Evening Session

Reflect on your day and now write 5 things or people that you are grateful for! Be Specific about your day. Remember you can be grateful for people, yourself or objects.

1. _____

   _____

2. _____

   _____

3. _____

   _____

4. _____

   _____

5. _____

   _____

Has it been a hard day? This is where you write 5 things or people you want to forgive. Again, do not forget to be specific about the day! And remember you can include yourself, people or objects.

1. _____

   _____

2. _____

   _____

3. _____

   _____

4. _____

   _____

5. _____

   _____

Reflection Space

This is your space! This is where you can make a few notes, you can do a spider diagram, you can doodle, or you can simply write down how you feel. If you are going to write down how you feel, remember to not rant and whine about your day, but to think of about, what you have learnt from the day and how you could improve for the next day. Ranting and moaning about the day will only create negative emotions and leave you feeling down. Keep it positive!

FRIDAY

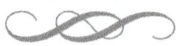

Morning Session

Find a quote, lyric, a picture, or something you have heard and stick it underneath. This is what you are going to start your day with! Make it funny or positive. Just as long as it makes you feel good. It is your dandelion in the concreate for the day!

Now write 5 goals that you want to achieve today. Remember you can make them small, medium or big, but make them achievable! Do not write things that you will not be able to achieve and whatever you cannot complete today does not roll over to tomorrow.

1. _____

   _____

2. _____

   _____

3. _____

   _____

4. _____

   _____

5. _____

   _____

Evening Session

Reflect on your day and now write 5 things or people that you are grateful for! Be Specific about your day. Remember you can be grateful for people, yourself or objects.

1. _____

   _____

2. _____

   _____

3. _____

   _____

4. _____

   _____

5. _____

   _____

Has it been a hard day? This is where you write 5 things or people you want to forgive. Again, do not forget to be specific about the day! And remember you can include yourself, people or objects.

1. _____

   _____

2. _____

   _____

3. _____

   _____

4. _____

   _____

5. _____

   _____

Reflection Space

This is your space! This is where you can make a few notes, you can do a spider diagram, you can doodle, or you can simply write down how you feel. If you are going to write down how you feel, remember to not rant and whine about your day, but to think of about, what you have learnt from the day and how you could improve for the next day. Ranting and moaning about the day will only create negative emotions and leave you feeling down. Keep it positive!

SATURDAY

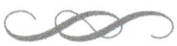

Morning Session

Find a quote, lyric, a picture, or something you have heard and stick it underneath. This is what you are going to start your day with! Make it funny or positive. Just as long as it makes you feel good. It is your dandelion in the concreate for the day!

Now write 5 goals that you want to achieve today. Remember you can make them small, medium or big, but make them achievable! Do not write things that you will not be able to achieve and whatever you cannot complete today does not roll over to tomorrow.

1. _____

   _____

2. _____

   _____

3. _____

   _____

4. _____

   _____

5. _____

   _____

Evening Session

Reflect on your day and now write 5 things or people that you are grateful for! Be Specific about your day. Remember you can be grateful for people, yourself or objects.

1. _____

   _____

2. _____

   _____

3. _____

   _____

4. _____

   _____

5. _____

   _____

Has it been a hard day? This is where you write 5 things or people you want to forgive. Again, do not forget to be specific about the day! And remember you can include yourself, people or objects.

1. _____

   _____

2. _____

   _____

3. _____

   _____

4. _____

   _____

5. _____

   _____

Reflection Space

This is your space! This is where you can make a few notes, you can do a spider diagram, you can doodle, or you can simply write down how you feel. If you are going to write down how you feel, remember to not rant and whine about your day, but to think of about, what you have learnt from the day and how you could improve for the next day. Ranting and moaning about the day will only create negative emotions and leave you feeling down. Keep it positive!

SUNDAY

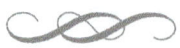

Morning Session

Find a quote, lyric, a picture, or something you have heard and stick it underneath. This is what you are going to start your day with! Make it funny or positive. Just as long as it makes you feel good. It is your dandelion in the concreate for the day!

Now write 5 goals that you want to achieve today. Remember you can make them small, medium or big, but make them achievable! Do not write things that you will not be able to achieve and whatever you cannot complete today does not roll over to tomorrow.

1. _____

   _____

2. _____

   _____

3. _____

   _____

4. _____

   _____

5. _____

   _____

Evening Session

Reflect on your day and now write 5 things or people that you are grateful for! Be Specific about your day. Remember you can be grateful for people, yourself or objects.

1. _____

   _____

2. _____

   _____

3. _____

   _____

4. _____

   _____

5. _____

   _____

Has it been a hard day? This is where you write 5 things or people you want to forgive. Again, do not forget to be specific about the day! And remember you can include yourself, people or objects.

1. _____

_____

2. _____

_____

3. _____

_____

4. _____

_____

5. _____

_____

Reflection Space

This is your space! This is where you can make a few notes, you can do a spider diagram, you can doodle, or you can simply write down how you feel. If you are going to write down how you feel, remember to not rant and whine about your day, but to think of about, what you have learnt from the day and how you could improve for the next day. Ranting and moaning about the day will only create negative emotions and leave you feeling down. Keep it positive!

HEAL YOURSELF

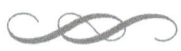

In Ancient Chinese philosophy they have the yin and yang which is a concept of dualism, describing how opposite forces compliment each other and how they interrelate to one another. The yin is known to be the darkness and the yang is known to be the lightness. Without one, the other can not exist nor can it be balanced, so how does this apply to us? In life, we have to have darkness to appreciate the light and with light, we have darkness, but it is how we heal from the darkness that matters.

There is no doubt that some people are better at self-healing than others. They have in built resilience, and it can appear that they have superhuman strength to just keep going, but what it is about those people that helps them to keep moving forward.

The most important difference is that the self-healer believes in the power of the mind. They do not just hope it is going to work; they believe it's going to work. There is a clear connection between the way your mind thinks and the way your body feels. you can also use your mind to improve your body, simply by changing the way you think and taking charge of what occupies your mind and while positive thinking won't cure everything, a healthy mindset is a key component to a healthy body.

Another thing that self-healers are exceptionally good at doing is that they treat themselves in a kind, gentle and supportive way as if they were treating a loved one in need. If you were going to give the same support to someone in need, then why are you not giving yourself, the same love, care and compassion? Why do you feel it is ok to be hard on yourself and to not give yourself the time that you need to heal? Why do you have such high expectations on yourself?

Maybe it is time to drop all those expectations that you have put on yourself over the years, all the conditions that people and society have put on you and look to yourself! Look to what you what you want to do in life and look at how you want to be? Be kind to yourself. Be compassionate to yourself. Learn who you are and learn to love who you are without no judgements or conditions and learn to be free!

MONDAY

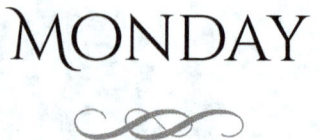

Morning Session

Find a quote, lyric, a picture, or something you have heard and stick it underneath. This is what you are going to start your day with! Make it funny or positive. Just as long as it makes you feel good. It is your dandelion in the concreate for the day!

Now write 5 goals that you want to achieve today. Remember you can make them small, medium or big, but make them achievable! Do not write things that you will not be able to achieve and whatever you cannot complete today does not roll over to tomorrow.

1. _____

   _____

2. _____

   _____

3. _____

   _____

4. _____

   _____

5. _____

   _____

Evening Session

Reflect on your day and now write 5 things or people that you are grateful for! Be Specific about your day. Remember you can be grateful for people, yourself or objects.

1. _____

   _____

2. _____

   _____

3. _____

   _____

4. _____

   _____

5. _____

   _____

Has it been a hard day? This is where you write 5 things or people you want to forgive. Again, do not forget to be specific about the day! And remember you can include yourself, people or objects.

1. _____
   _____

2. _____
   _____

3. _____
   _____

4. _____
   _____

5. _____
   _____

Reflection Space

This is your space! This is where you can make a few notes, you can do a spider diagram, you can doodle, or you can simply write down how you feel. If you are going to write down how you feel, remember to not rant and whine about your day, but to think of about, what you have learnt from the day and how you could improve for the next day. Ranting and moaning about the day will only create negative emotions and leave you feeling down. Keep it positive!

TUESDAY

Morning Session

Find a quote, lyric, a picture, or something you have heard and stick it underneath. This is what you are going to start your day with! Make it funny or positive. Just as long as it makes you feel good. It is your dandelion in the concreate for the day!

Now write 5 goals that you want to achieve today. Remember you can make them small, medium or big, but make them achievable! Do not write things that you will not be able to achieve and whatever you cannot complete today does not roll over to tomorrow.

1. _____

   _____

2. _____

   _____

3. _____

   _____

4. _____

   _____

5. _____

   _____

Evening Session

Reflect on your day and now write 5 things or people that you are grateful for! Be Specific about your day. Remember you can be grateful for people, yourself or objects.

1. _____

_____

2. _____

_____

3. _____

_____

4. _____

_____

5. _____

_____

Has it been a hard day? This is where you write 5 things or people you want to forgive. Again, do not forget to be specific about the day! And remember you can include yourself, people or objects.

1. _____

   _____

2. _____

   _____

3. _____

   _____

4. _____

   _____

5. _____

   _____

Reflection Space

This is your space! This is where you can make a few notes, you can do a spider diagram, you can doodle, or you can simply write down how you feel. If you are going to write down how you feel, remember to not rant and whine about your day, but to think of about, what you have learnt from the day and how you could improve for the next day. Ranting and moaning about the day will only create negative emotions and leave you feeling down. Keep it positive!

WEDNESDAY

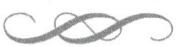

Morning Session

Find a quote, lyric, a picture, or something you have heard and stick it underneath. This is what you are going to start your day with! Make it funny or positive. Just as long as it makes you feel good. It is your dandelion in the concreate for the day!

Now write 5 goals that you want to achieve today. Remember you can make them small, medium or big, but make them achievable! Do not write things that you will not be able to achieve and whatever you cannot complete today does not roll over to tomorrow.

1. _____

   _____

2. _____

   _____

3. _____

   _____

4. _____

   _____

5. _____

   _____

Evening Session

Reflect on your day and now write 5 things or people that you are grateful for! Be Specific about your day. Remember you can be grateful for people, yourself or objects.

1. _____

_____

2. _____

_____

3. _____

_____

4. _____

_____

5. _____

_____

Has it been a hard day? This is where you write 5 things or people you want to forgive. Again, do not forget to be specific about the day! And remember you can include yourself, people or objects.

1. _____

   _____

2. _____

   _____

3. _____

   _____

4. _____

   _____

5. _____

   _____

Reflection Space

This is your space! This is where you can make a few notes, you can do a spider diagram, you can doodle, or you can simply write down how you feel. If you are going to write down how you feel, remember to not rant and whine about your day, but to think of about, what you have learnt from the day and how you could improve for the next day. Ranting and moaning about the day will only create negative emotions and leave you feeling down. Keep it positive!

THURSDAY

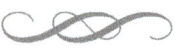

Morning Session

Find a quote, lyric, a picture, or something you have heard and stick it underneath. This is what you are going to start your day with! Make it funny or positive. Just as long as it makes you feel good. It is your dandelion in the concreate for the day!

Now write 5 goals that you want to achieve today. Remember you can make them small, medium or big, but make them achievable! Do not write things that you will not be able to achieve and whatever you cannot complete today does not roll over to tomorrow.

1. _____

   _____

2. _____

   _____

3. _____

   _____

4. _____

   _____

5. _____

   _____

Evening Session

Reflect on your day and now write 5 things or people that you are grateful for! Be Specific about your day. Remember you can be grateful for people, yourself or objects.

1. _____

   _____

2. _____

   _____

3. _____

   _____

4. _____

   _____

5. _____

   _____

Has it been a hard day? This is where you write 5 things or people you want to forgive. Again, do not forget to be specific about the day! And remember you can include yourself, people or objects.

1. _____

   _____

2. _____

   _____

3. _____

   _____

4. _____

   _____

5. _____

   _____

Reflection Space

This is your space! This is where you can make a few notes, you can do a spider diagram, you can doodle, or you can simply write down how you feel. If you are going to write down how you feel, remember to not rant and whine about your day, but to think of about, what you have learnt from the day and how you could improve for the next day. Ranting and moaning about the day will only create negative emotions and leave you feeling down. Keep it positive!

FRIDAY

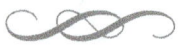

Morning Session

Find a quote, lyric, a picture, or something you have heard and stick it underneath. This is what you are going to start your day with! Make it funny or positive. Just as long as it makes you feel good. It is your dandelion in the concreate for the day!

Now write 5 goals that you want to achieve today. Remember you can make them small, medium or big, but make them achievable! Do not write things that you will not be able to achieve and whatever you cannot complete today does not roll over to tomorrow.

1. _____

   _____

2. _____

   _____

3. _____

   _____

4. _____

   _____

5. _____

   _____

Evening Session

Reflect on your day and now write 5 things or people that you are grateful for! Be Specific about your day. Remember you can be grateful for people, yourself or objects.

1. _____

   _____

2. _____

   _____

3. _____

   _____

4. _____

   _____

5. _____

   _____

Has it been a hard day? This is where you write 5 things or people you want to forgive. Again, do not forget to be specific about the day! And remember you can include yourself, people or objects.

1. _____

_____

2. _____

_____

3. _____

_____

4. _____

_____

5. _____

_____

Reflection Space

This is your space! This is where you can make a few notes, you can do a spider diagram, you can doodle, or you can simply write down how you feel. If you are going to write down how you feel, remember to not rant and whine about your day, but to think of about, what you have learnt from the day and how you could improve for the next day. Ranting and moaning about the day will only create negative emotions and leave you feeling down. Keep it positive!

SATURDAY

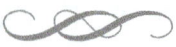

Morning Session

Find a quote, lyric, a picture, or something you have heard and stick it underneath. This is what you are going to start your day with! Make it funny or positive. Just as long as it makes you feel good. It is your dandelion in the concreate for the day!

Now write 5 goals that you want to achieve today. Remember you can make them small, medium or big, but make them achievable! Do not write things that you will not be able to achieve and whatever you cannot complete today does not roll over to tomorrow.

1. _____

   _____

2. _____

   _____

3. _____

   _____

4. _____

   _____

5. _____

   _____

Evening Session

Reflect on your day and now write 5 things or people that you are grateful for! Be Specific about your day. Remember you can be grateful for people, yourself or objects.

1. _____

   _____

2. _____

   _____

3. _____

   _____

4. _____

   _____

5. _____

   _____

Has it been a hard day? This is where you write 5 things or people you want to forgive. Again, do not forget to be specific about the day! And remember you can include yourself, people or objects.

1. _____
   _____

2. _____
   _____

3. _____
   _____

4. _____
   _____

5. _____
   _____

Reflection Space

This is your space! This is where you can make a few notes, you can do a spider diagram, you can doodle, or you can simply write down how you feel. If you are going to write down how you feel, remember to not rant and whine about your day, but to think of about, what you have learnt from the day and how you could improve for the next day. Ranting and moaning about the day will only create negative emotions and leave you feeling down. Keep it positive!

SUNDAY

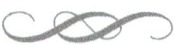

Morning Session

Find a quote, lyric, a picture, or something you have heard and stick it underneath. This is what you are going to start your day with! Make it funny or positive. Just as long as it makes you feel good. It is your dandelion in the concreate for the day!

Now write 5 goals that you want to achieve today. Remember you can make them small, medium or big, but make them achievable! Do not write things that you will not be able to achieve and whatever you cannot complete today does not roll over to tomorrow.

1. _____

   _____

2. _____

   _____

3. _____

   _____

4. _____

   _____

5. _____

   _____

Evening Session

Reflect on your day and now write 5 things or people that you are grateful for! Be Specific about your day. Remember you can be grateful for people, yourself or objects.

1. _____

   _____

2. _____

   _____

3. _____

   _____

4. _____

   _____

5. _____

   _____

Has it been a hard day? This is where you write 5 things or people you want to forgive. Again, do not forget to be specific about the day! And remember you can include yourself, people or objects.

1. _____

   _____

2. _____

   _____

3. _____

   _____

4. _____

   _____

5. _____

   _____

Reflection Space

This is your space! This is where you can make a few notes, you can do a spider diagram, you can doodle, or you can simply write down how you feel. If you are going to write down how you feel, remember to not rant and whine about your day, but to think of about, what you have learnt from the day and how you could improve for the next day. Ranting and moaning about the day will only create negative emotions and leave you feeling down. Keep it positive!

LETTING GO

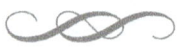

Most people have the same goal in life, which is that they want to feel happy. Yet in order to be happy we have to put ourselves in the frontline of pain and at times, get hurt. For some people, this pain can leave an imprint into their lives which can affect them every day. Eckhart Tolle believes that we create and maintain our own problems because they give us a sense of identity. This could explain why some of us hold onto our pain a lot longer than we need to.

We sometimes pin our happiness on to people, circumstances and things in the hope that this will make us happy and hold on them, often losing sight of where we are currently and where we want to go. In holding on to what is familiar, we often limit ourselves by not allowing ourselves to experience the present or think about what may come next, this is why it is important to let go. Letting go is no simple task and can be a commitment in itself, but there are certain things we can practice.

Live in each moment. Do not try to look backwards or forwards. Focus on what is happening then and remember, that whether it is good or bad, it will not last forever. Nothing is permanent and trying to fight this, will only cause you pain in the future. Life is fluid, learn to let it go.

We are nature's children, and we grow the way a plant grows, from a seed to a bud to a plant. You will not be the same at any given moment. You will be moving, growing and evolving as a person. Give yourself the flexibility and space to grow and develop and give others around you to do the same. Remember that you cannot control at what pace others grow and develop, you can only support them.

Know that the past is the past, and you will not be able to change or control it. We can only understand it and work towards for forgiveness. The only way to relieve your pain is to accept what has happened in the past and leave it in the past. Be replaying past events over and over again in our head and allowing feelings of pain and hurt shape our actions in the present will only cause us more pain and health issues.

When we accept responsibility for our experiences and feelings, we learn that we have more control over our lives than what we thought.

We cannot control what happens in the world around us, but we can choose how we interpret and interact with it and letting go and forgiving the past is a great way to start.

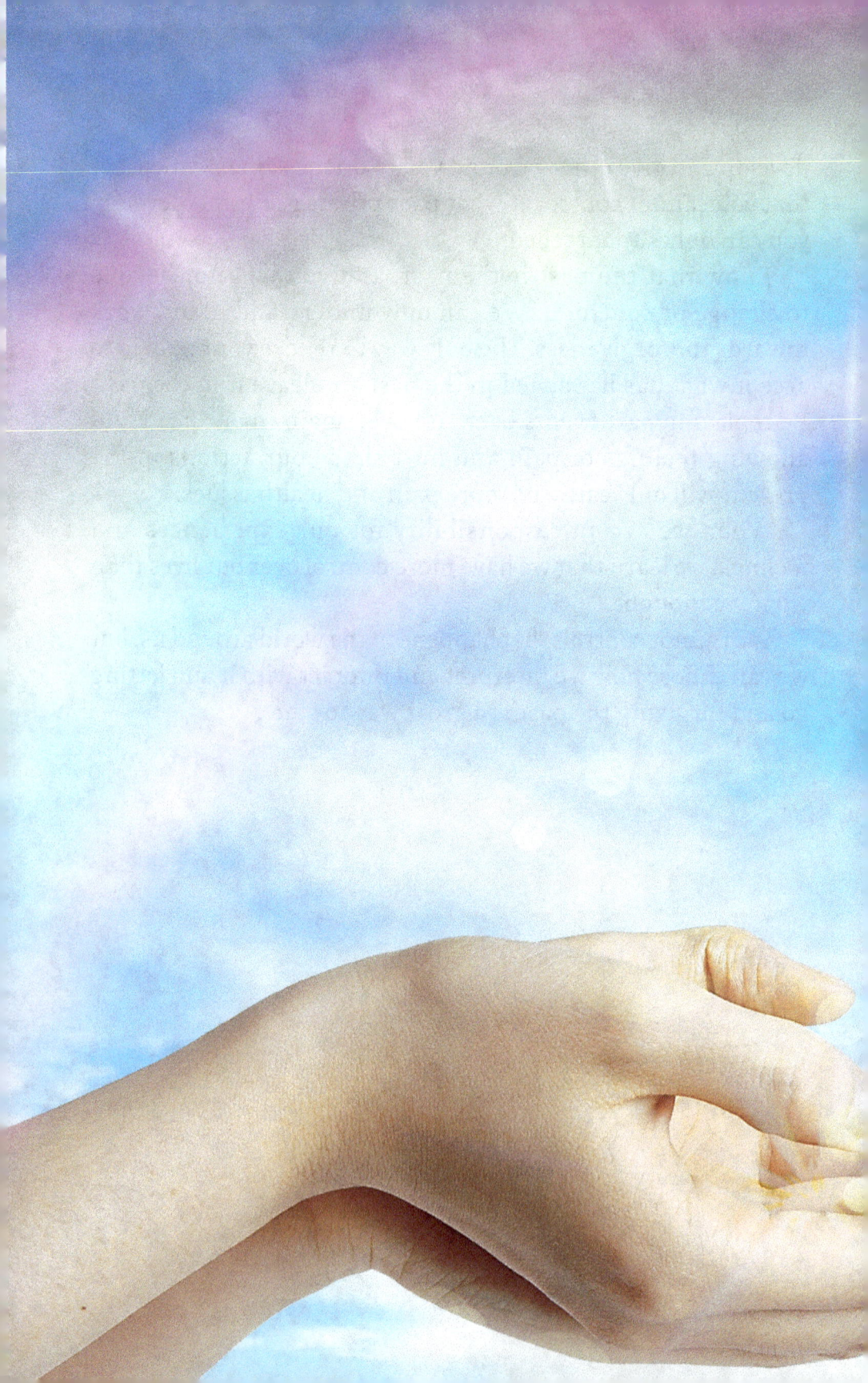

MY NOTE TO YOU!

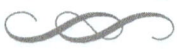

Well done! You should now give yourself a pat on the back and do something to celebrate as you have now finished the 12 weeks programme. Looking back over the 12 weeks, ask yourself the following questions.

Can you write down five things that the Journal has helped you to discover about yourself?

1. _____

2. _____

3. _____

4. _____

5. _____

You will have learnt a lot of new skills over the 12-week period such as learning to be patience with yourself, showing gratitude in everyday life and being able to reflect on positive events. Take some time and
Celebrate all what you have learned and embrace it. Praise the things that you have learned about yourself, as you can only grow and develop this as you move forward with your life.

List five things that you have implemented in your life to better yourself every day?

1. _____
   _____

2. _____
   _____

3. _____
   _____

4. _____
   _____

5. _____
   _____

It is a positive start that you have made where you have begun to implement changes in your life for the better. However, it is important to remember that anything we want to implement, we now really need to concentrate on practicing and learning how to really embed these ideas and beliefs in our lives every day for them to be maintained. Really think about how you are going to do this and maybe think about the barriers that may get in the way of embedding these ideas and beliefs, so that you can be better prepare for it. Try to remember that these changes are not just for one day or for a week but for a lifetime. They should flow naturally every day and on the days that they do not flow so easily, practice forgiveness and acceptance with yourself.

Every day, It is important to practice self-appreciation as well, by acknowledging the positive within you without the need to compare yourself to others and be grateful for the things and people around you.

List five things that you feel you still need to work on to help you reach your goal of being positive every day?

1. _____
   _____

2. _____
   _____

3. _____
   _____

4. _____
   _____

5. _____
   _____

Even though you have worked so hard in the 12 weeks, there will still be some things that you want to work on and achieve. Being happy is a full-time commitment and there will always be things you might want to work on to get a better you. Do not see this as a bad thing, see it as a positive thing. Remember we are always growing and developing all the time and as people we are fluid and never stagnant.

Remember that happiness comes from within. Learn to tame the negative

thoughts and approach every day with optimism. As a result, you will reach your end goal of being happy and achieving inner peace.

Keep striving for better and never give up. Even the small steps that we take will lead you somewhere and eventually you will end up where you need to be.

There are no limits to what you can now accomplish, start focusing on what is present and appreciate your life.

ABOUT THE AUTHOR

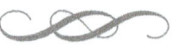

MY VISION

Hi, my name is Kruti St Helen and I really believe that life is about learning and growth. I really want to pass on the message to people to embrace life and to not be scared of failing and really commit yourself to personal growth and development, but have fun doing it.

ABOUT ME

I am a qualified Accredited Counsellor/Psychotherapist and a Counselling Tutor with over fifteen years of experience. I was born and raised in the East End of London, and then I moved down to the South of England, near the beach. I love being by the sea and love going out for walks and being outdoors. I love travelling and enjoy embracing various cultures, and travel a lot with my family.

EXPERIENCE

I have worked with a diverse range of people in many different organisations. Currently I provide long and short-term counselling sessions, providing face to face, online and telephone counselling using an integrative model, drawing on skills from CBT, Solution Focused Therapy, Gestalt and Person Centred. I work with adults, adolescents, and children conducting play therapy, and with couples.

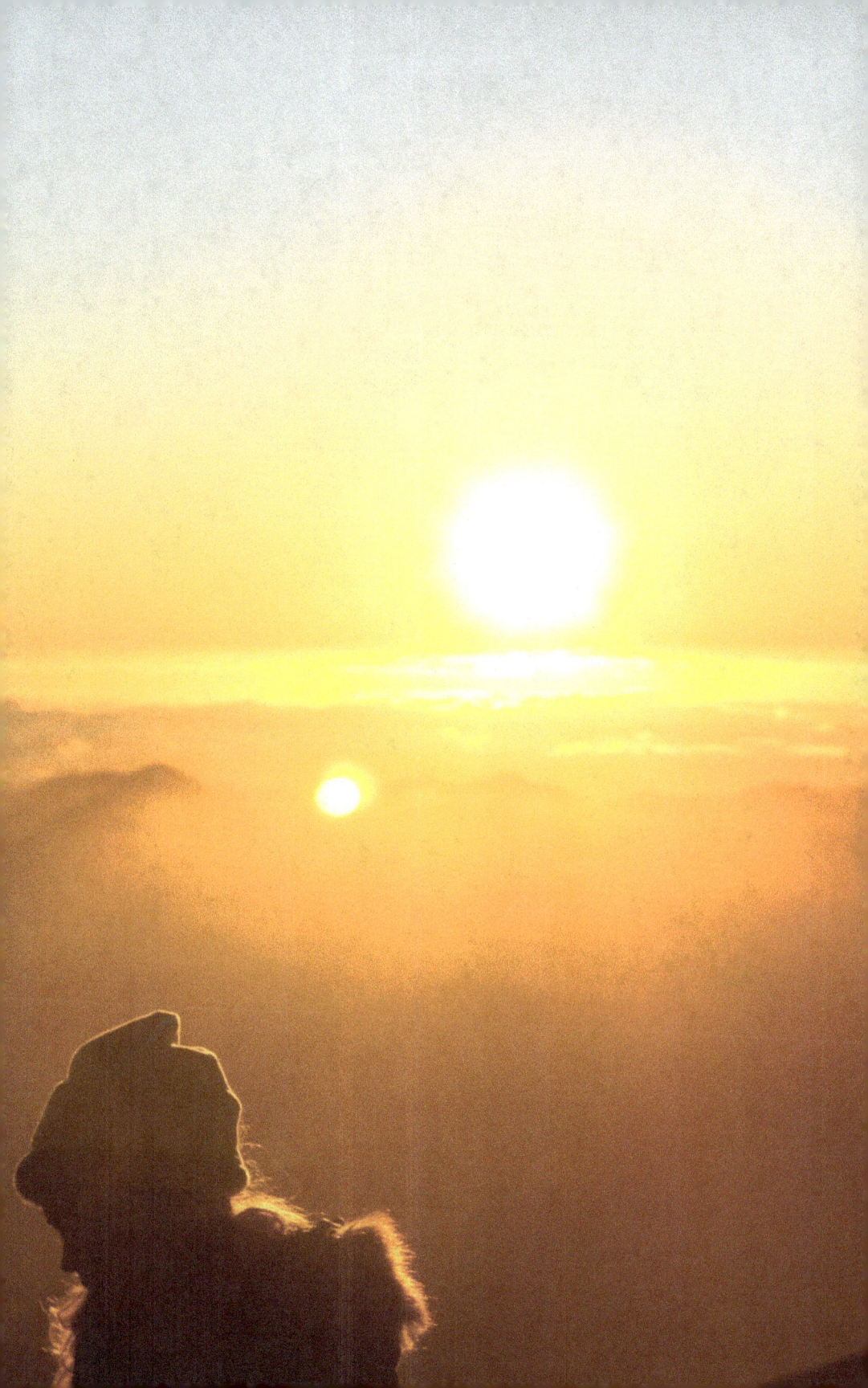

www.ingramcontent.com/pod-product-compliance
Lightning Source LLC
Chambersburg PA
CBHW071801080526
44589CB00012B/631